RED MIRACLE

RED MIRACLE

The Story of Soviet Medicine

By EDWARD PODOLSKY, M.D.

Woodcut Illustrations by Hans Alexander Mueller

Essay Index Reprint Series

BOOKS FOR LIBRARIES PRESS
FREEPORT, NEW YORK

Dedicated To

JEFFREY

Library of Congress Cataloging in Publication Data

Podolsky, Edward, 1902-
  Red miracle.

  (Essay index reprint series)
  Bibliography: p.
  1. Medicine--Russia--History. 2. Medicine,
State--Russia. I. Title.
[R531.P6 1972]   610'.947   70-167402
ISBN 0-8369-2818-0

PRINTED IN THE UNITED STATES OF AMERICA
BY
NEW WORLD BOOK MANUFACTURING CO., INC.
HALLANDALE, FLORIDA 33009

CONTENTS

8　　　　　　　　　　CONTENTS

Part Three

A GALLERY OF RUSSIAN DOCTORS

Part Four

THE PROMISE OF THE FUTURE

(Halftone illustrations follow p. 98 in text.)

FOREWORD

MOST books written on Soviet medicine lack universality and details. Dr. Podolsky in his book, *Red Miracle,* fills in these gaps. He enlightens his readers with biographical data on Soviet medical pioneers, as well as their successes in the field of medicine in the Soviet Union.

The word "miracle" does not carry the usual symbolism, but here applies to real progress that was achieved by the tireless efforts of scientific workers, public as well as government employees, who worked as a team in combating the diseases that for centuries were rampant in the country.

The statistical data given in *Red Miracle* are vivid proof of the colossal achievements in the field of medicine since 1918.

Soviet medicine began from the first day of the October Revolution. The scientists, conscious of their responsibilities, disregarding all difficulties and obstacles that confronted them, worked tirelessly to combat disease and for the improvement of public welfare.

The Russian scientists began to work on the ruins left from World War I, blockades, civil war, and intervention. They kept on fighting against all kinds of contagious diseases and epidemics. But for this, they needed equipment and trained personnel. The government with the help of trade unions and local organizations established numerous clinics, health centers, sanatoria, hospitals. and medical universities in all parts of the country. In the universities priority was given to the students from the rural districts. After graduation they willingly returned to their own homes in the capacities in which they were trained. Most of them were physicians. The

9

struggle was directed along two paths: one was for the elimination of disease, and the second for the prevention of disease. Much emphasis is laid on preventive medicine. Periodical check-up on the health of school children is a known fact. They established numerous kindergartens, rest homes and hygiene centers. With these, they made tremendous strides in the improvement of health and sanitation. A program was instituted for the education of the people through books, pamphlets, newspapers, lectures and moving pictures.

The medical achievements of the Soviet Union would have been nullified without progress made in other fields, such as education, industry, transportation, and agriculture. All these problems were tackled by the Soviet people with the same strength. They disregarded personal comfort, and were willing to sacrifice whatever they had in their possession for the eradication of what was old, and for building a new country.

As a graduate of Saratov University, I take pride in being a student of Professor A. A. Bogomolets, who made himself immortal with his discovery of the method of blood banking, and Anti-Reticular Cytotoxic Serum (A.C.S.). It was a "miracle" that Professor Bogomolets made dying people walk with blood of cadavers circulating through their bodies, or hoped to extend our life-span for 150 years with the help of the A.C.S. serum.

Professor Spasokukatski, also a teacher of mine, invented a formula for "feeding" patients, who had undergone an abdominal operation, directly through the intestines. Thanks to his method, the percentage of casualties from abdominal operations was greatly reduced.

Professor N. A. Bogoraz of Rostov-on-the-Don University, made short people happy by lengthening the bones of their lower extremities, thereby increasing their height. One of the bigger tasks that he tackled is curing people popularly known as "midgets" of their dwarfish stature. Midgets, in whom the gland which regulates growth has been missing from birth, settle down in the clinic until a gland for transplanting is available from a dead person of normal height. It was the professor himself who held a congress of surgeons and physicians of the Azov and Black Sea regions spellbound with his daring demonstration of how surgical intervention can create a brand-new functioning organ. The large gathering of specialists was visibly shaken when Bogoraz cut two striplets from the body of the patient who had lost his sex organ, and from the two created a new living, normally functioning organ. After the operation, the patient became a father.

Reading Dr. Podolsky's *Red Miracle* gives me a clear idea of the progress that has been made in the field of medicine. I was working in the district of Karayas, Caucasus, where malaria has been prevalent for many centuries. A proverb existed in this district: "Malaria kills like flies, and those who have no malaria are illegitimate children." The people were so used to malaria that they had lost all hope of getting well. The Soviet government used every means to exterminate malaria, including drainage of stagnant water, filling of swamps, and pouring kerosene on stagnant water where drainage was impossible. In two years there was a tremendous improvement in the elimination of malaria. For centuries, the population was kept in ignorance, and, for lack of physicians, they became easy prey for the witch doctors. One night, I was roused from sleep by a loud and excited voice, saying, "Our cow is expecting a calf." When I resented this "insult" the man replied: "Well, the other day you helped my neighbor's wife, why don't you help my cow?" On another occasion, I was called in to attend an eight-year-old boy who had a high fever and was in a state of delirium. I was shocked when I saw that his back was furrowed with numerous incisions made by the razor of a witch doctor with the idea of letting the evil spirits out of his body. The boy was suffering from pneumonia. The president of the local soviet advised me not to remove the boy to the local hospital. He said: "He is half dead. If he dies in hospital you will be blamed for it. You don't know our people. They will kill you." Despite this warning and interference, I removed the boy to the hospital. Fortunately, he recovered. On another occasion, I was called in to attend a woman who had just given birth to a dead child. She was sitting on the ashes in a stable with the cows. The purpose of the ashes was to stop hemorrhage. She was in an appalling state, feverish, and delirious. She was immediately removed to our hospital. An old woman told me: "Doctor, don't take her to the hospital, her placenta was stolen by a ghost, and she never will recover." Ignoring ghost and old woman, she was removed to the hospital, where she recovered uneventfully.

The struggle between myself and the witch doctor grew keener. I was warned to leave the district or to be prepared to meet the consequences. I remained in the district and was ready to meet the consequences with a pistol in my pocket.

Red Miracle is an authentic source of information which Dr. Podolsky acquired through his tireless study of the medical situation in the Soviet Union. His book is a valid document that should be read by every unbiased truth-seeker, and by men from every walk of life. In writing on Soviet medicine, Dr. Podolsky indirectly has touched on every branch of social life in that country, and proves that the *Red Miracle* is actually a Red reality.

PAUL G. EDGAR, M.D.

New York City.

INTRODUCTION

S OCIALIZED medicine is in the news today and has been for quite some time. Many people have a nebulous idea as to what socialized medicine is and does. They have heard many arguments for and against it, and have a faint notion that it is practiced on the largest scale in the Soviet Union. That is true. Socialized medicine is the *only* kind of medicine practiced in the U.S.S.R. today.

How do people live under socialized or government medicine? What are the benefits they derive? What kind of doctors are produced under this system? Are they good doctors or poor ones? Can medical research flourish, and if so, what kind of medical science does this system produce?

In this book I have attempted to answer these questions. I have attempted to tell the story of socialized medicine in Russia without bias or prejudice. There is also a fascinating story to relate regarding medical research in Russia today, and this also I have attempted in this volume. I think that Russian medical sociology and research are two vital and interesting subjects about which everyone should know, for many of the Russian experiments and achievements are destined to shape the course medical science will follow in the future.

In writing this book I have leaned heavily upon the *American Review of Soviet Medicine,* official organ of the American-Soviet Medical Society, of which I am a member. The library of this society is a veritable treasure-house of Soviet medical literature, and I am most grateful for the aid which was so cordially extended me while engaged in research on the present volume. The *American Review of Soviet*

Medicine, a bi-monthly publication, presents original articles by American authorities on Russian medicine, as well as by Soviet medical men, whose writings are competently translated from the Russian. For those of my readers who are interested in the constantly progressive picture of Russian medical sociology and research this periodical should be consulted regularly.

The battle, centering about the introduction of some form of socialized medicine in this country, has been long and bitter. It is destined to become more so. This book attempts no more than to reveal the shape of socialized medicine in the only country where it is practiced on a gigantic, nation-wide scale, in the hope that the American public will be able at least to learn the truth behind the headlines, and judge for themselves.

EDWARD PODOLSKY, M.D.

Brooklyn, New York.

Part One

THE PRACTICE OF MEDICINE
IN THE SOVIET UNION

I

THE BEGINNINGS OF SOVIET MEDICINE

THE odor of decay stretched like a cloud across the land, from the western border to the farthest reaches of Siberia. The Czarist regime was breathing its last. A corrupt and feudal society was trying vainly to retain a strangle-hold grip on the people, and these final days were characterized by almost unbelievable depths of human misery and suffering. Living conditions of the workers in the cities, the peasants and farm laborers in the country, were vile. The police were everywhere; they had put into force vicious restrictive measures which bound the populace hand and foot. The dread word, "Siberia," acted as a whip to keep the people docile and subdued.

The laborers and peasants were hardly recognized as human beings with human desires, feelings and rights. The rich, feudal land owners, the quasi-fascistic army, the industrialists exploited them mercilessly. The general cultural level of the population was low and was deliberately kept low, for, as every despot knew, thinking and reading and hoping for a better life always led to trouble.

The medical profession during these dark days of the last Czar was in a pathetic state. The country was unequipped to combat the epidemic diseases which were becoming altogether too frequent. There were too few doctors, too few medical dispensaries, too few hospitals. In fact, many large cities and even provinces were totally lacking in physicians and medical supplies. For instance, huge territories which now form the autonomous republics of Kirghizia, Chuvashia

17

and Uzbekistan were left entirely without doctors. Hygienic conditions were extremely bad. Superstition and ignorance helped the spread of diseases, especially those that were infectious. The annual toll of lives was in the millions.

It is difficult to obtain a complete statistical analysis of the spread of diseases during the Czarist regime because vital and other statistics were very badly kept. What figures we do possess are unreliable. Yet it is known that of all diseases, one-fourth were due directly to poor economic and living conditions. Lack of knowledge, lack of proper equipment, lack of sanitary precautions caused typhus and typhoid fever to rage throughout the vast territories and kill a half million people in the short space of a single decade. At the same time, smallpox claimed its hundreds of thousands of lives. Plague epidemics were common. The records indicate that millions of lives were snuffed out by diseases which could have been prevented by the application of but a few sanitary rules. There is no doubt that the number who suffered and died was much greater since many deaths as the result of a specific disease were never reported. The peasants, feeling ill, would often not trouble to seek medical aid, particularly as the nearest medical station was usually some twenty miles away, and twenty miles is a long distance to walk when you have a debilitating fever.

The story of Czarist Russia is a shameful story in the medical history of mankind. It is a story of carelessness, brutality and sheer disinterest, where an easily avoidable disease such as trachoma was allowed to take its toll of man's happiness and well-being simply because it was too much trouble to educate the people to take a few elementary precautions. Trachoma, an epidemic eye disease, was so widespread that it blinded hundreds of thousands of human beings needlessly; a few simple hygienic rules would have enabled these blinded people to retain their sight. As a result, Czarist Russia had the dubious distinction of leading the world in the number of blind inhabitants. Human life was cheap; it was sacrificed for trifles. Stupidity, superstition and ignorance maimed, crippled and killed.

As an example of what superstition and ignorance could do in the spread of disease and suffering, consider the spread of syphilis through non-sexual contact, such as kissing, eating from a common dish and nursing children. Entire villages, districts and provinces were affected by this disease. It was as common as a cold. So widespread were the effects of this disease that many villages in the Russia of the "Little Father" were known as *Kurnosovka* (snub-nose). Snub-nose is a common characteristic of the ravages of syphilis. Very often in the tertiary stage of the disease the bridge of the nose is eaten away, causing the nose to collapse and creating a snub or saddle-like indentation. But this will happen only when the disease is untreated and neglected. In the cities, syphilis constituted 35 per cent of all diseases, while in the outlying districts this figure often reached as high as 65 per cent of the total.

The science of pediatrics—the care and treatment of children—was unknown in Czarist Russia. Child mortality was extremely high. A child was born under unhygienic conditions, was cared for amid primitive surroundings, subjected to poor nutritional management, contracted one of the numerous childhood infections. With characteristic Russian resignation not much was done. A child was born, lived a brief time and died. Soon another child was born, was fortunate in avoiding disease and lived. The Lord gave and the Lord took away, and there was not much that one could do about it. Medical science was primitive and what there was of it was not for the peasant, the worker, the humble citizen. It also goes without saying that the general rate of mortality was exceptionally high.

Things were not getting better with the passing of the years; if anything, they were getting worse. Let us quote

Dr. N. A. Semashko, who became the first People's Commissar of Health in 1918: "With the outbreak of war the picture became even more gloomy. The general economic conditions, and consequently the sanitary conditions, of the population, became still worse. Mass migrations (war refugees, war prisoners, soldiers on leave) promoted the spread of infection to which the weakened human organism became particularly susceptible. Terrible war losses (it has been calculated that Russia had nearly twenty million killed and disabled during World War I) in turn dealt a staggering blow to the country. On the other hand, the medical service, poor as it was, was finally disorganized, the great majority of the doctors having been mobilized for the war. Owing to food, fuel and other difficulties, the lack of necessary medicines for the patients, even the hospitals which remained intact dragged on to a miserable existence, while some were forced to close down.

"It is hardly necessary to say that no medical statistics of any value were kept at that time. One thing is clear, that the war completely undermined both the health of the population and the medical organization. The breakdown was complete.

"It was under such conditions that the Soviet power took over the health services. It was necessary to carry out a radical revolution in these services and to bring order out of chaos. It was necessary to reorganize the entire public health system both in the principles on which it was based, in its organization and in its principal aspects along entirely new lines."

Dr. Semashko was one of the really great and enlightened leaders of medical reform in the new Russia. His methods and ideas were regarded as so radical as to be impossible of achievement and met with some blind opposition from the old guard, the men who could not make too quick a change. But in the end, after a valiant struggle and an unceasing campaign to break down the barriers of prejudice and defeatist outlook, he won out. The few conservatives quickly saw that they were wrong and that Semashko was right. They came over wholeheartedly to his side and gave him the fullest support.

Dr. Semashko organized and put into effective operation the Narkomzdrav or the People's Commissariat of Health, of which he was the first head. Statistics, for the first time, were kept in a scientific and orderly fashion. Bacteriology, instead of dead house studies was emphasized. The trend was away from the academic to the vital, living functions of the human body. Measures of controlling and limiting infectious diseases were introduced and put into practice all over the country. The principles of personal and public hygiene were widely publicized.

Things were taking a turn for the better. Human life was acquiring a new dignity. The fight was now against disease and death with a vengeance. The People's Commissariat of Health was not the only new medical institution to be established during these early days of Soviet medicine. Other institutions were founded as well—the All-Union Institute of Experimental Medicine in Leningrad, with its branches, the Biological institutes in Moscow and Kharkov, the Tubercular institutes, the Venereological institutes, the Leningrad Institute of Physical Therapy, the Institute of Pathological Anatomy, the Labor Protection Institute, the Institute for the Study of Industrial Diseases, the Institute of Social Diseases, the Institute for the Study of Health Resorts, the Tropical Institute, the Physiological and Psychological Institute, and the Artificial Climate Pavilion. Somewhat later, a Leprosarium, considered one of the best in the world, was built in Holmsk, in the Crimean district. One can see from this impressive list of institutes how lusty was the rebirth of medicine in the newly organized and reborn land.

Contrasting sharply with the disinterest and inertia of the Czarist regime, one of the first measures taken by the Soviets was the organization of means and methods to protect and safeguard motherhood and childhood. The aim—to conserve life at its very source. A network of institutions and unions for the protection of children and mothers spread from one end of Russia to the other.

From Sherwood Eddy, an eminent American traveler and sociologist, who visited Russia in the early days of its rebirth, we learn that: "One of the most brilliant achievements of the Soviet Union is in the sphere of childhood and its attainment of free, compulsory, universal primary education. This is surprising to the newcomer in Russia, who would perhaps have expected in a revolutionary government a concentration upon material things and a more spartan rigor and even · neglect in dealing with childhood. Instead, it is as if the Revolution had taken a little child and set him in the midst of the whole system to occupy the first place of regard and almost of reverence. Children must be considered first in every law and plan. They must have the best milk, the most humane and scientific care, the chief consideration in everything. This is both instinctive and reflective. No people in the world have a greater natural wealth of affection for their children than the Russians, and no system gives more recognition to their importance. This is one evidence of the farsighted and enduring nature of the whole movement."

Another aspect of this problem is furnished in most illuminating terms by M. Vladimirsky, who, in his study of the public health problem, wrote: "To organize the life of millions of women who participate more and more in production and socialist construction—such is the problem at present which faces the organs of the Commissariat of Health in that particular section of work. This new problem changes also the methods of work. The work of protection of motherhood and infancy must be built as a mass work, which must satisfy the needs not of hundreds but of hundreds of thousands of working women."

As time went on, the movement to protect the health and

lives of the ordinary citizen gained in momentum. Health centers were founded everywhere in the Soviet republics. Each plant and factory had its own center in which to care for the health of the workers. Each district, each neighborhood, had its health organization for the instruction of the masses in matters regarding health, as well as for instituting practical measures for the control of disease.

A healthy and vigorous interest in medical research was manifested early in the Soviet republics and the network of medical research institutes, headed by the world-famous Institute of Experimental Medicine, contributed much to medical knowledge. Ivan Pavlov was the head of the Institute of Experimental Medicine in its early days. Pavlov was Russia's greatest physiologist even in the pre-Soviet period, but with the assumption of power by the Soviets his laboratory was brought up-to-date, new equipment was purchased and built, and working conditions improved immensely.

All of Soviet Russia became a beehive of healthful activity. During the years of the First and Second Five Year Plans, research in medical science went on at a constantly accelerated pace. New projects were put into execution. Additional laboratories and medical institutions were established everywhere. Unlimited funds were put at the disposal of research workers, physicians and medical scientists, and much valuable and important information was soon forthcoming along a dozen different frontiers of medical knowledge.

The primary and foremost aim of Soviet medicine was to make medical care available at all times to all the people. The very first Commissariat of Health began to socialize the entire process of medicine, in the hospitals and institutions, as well as among private physicians. Some opposition was encountered from the conservative elements of the medical profession in executing these plans, but soon this opposition melted away in the face of the obviously excellent results which were soon evident.

There is little doubt that Dr. Semashko will go down in medical history as one of the truly great medical leaders. His work as the first director of the Commissariat of Health was so outstanding that Lenin appointed him head of the State Department of Health. His greatest and most lasting accomplishment was the socialization of the practice of medicine. He was a man of great foresight, for it is his ideas which are now being recognized throughout the world, which are influencing countries far removed from Russia to regard government medicine favorably. Dr. Semashko was a tireless worker. After the conclusion of his labors for the state he devoted himself to a compilation of a *Cyclopedia of Medicine* which runs into more than forty volumes.

Dr. G. N. Kaminsky succeeded Semashko as Commissar of Health. During his administration the scope of the activities of his department increased greatly. He established many new dispensaries and clinics, particularly in the smaller towns and villages and in the most remote regions of the vast Russian republics. It was Dr. Kaminsky who introduced health insurance and insisted that every employer, whether a private entrepreneur or the government itself, carry insurance for all workers. Thus, universal health insurance became a reality for the first time.

With the increased interest in medicine and medical education, additional medical colleges were established throughout the new Russia. From the very beginning practical work was emphasized in medical education. The education of the medical student was thorough in every branch of medicine, including practical nursing.

Medical education, however, did not cease with graduation from medical school. Postgraduate work was encouraged by the Council of Medical Education. Special inducements were held out to young doctors up to thirty-five years of age. These physicians were enrolled in a selected aspirant group after they had passed examinations in special medical courses, natural sciences and foreign languages. The course of study was for three years; the first year was devoted to preclinical and theoretical consideration of the specialty being studied. After examinations in practical and theoretical studies, the aspirant, as he was known, devoted the rest of his course to clinical work in his specialty. Upon graduation he received a certificate rating him as a specialist in his particular field.

From the very beginning of the Soviet reorganization of the health facilities of the nation, all doctors were employed by the state and assigned to various medical, surgical and other types of institutions and hospitals according to their ability and experience. The desire to improve medical education, medical practice and medical research was manifested at all times, and effective measures were taken to bring this about.

The social and humanistic aspects of medical practice were not neglected. The two curses of Czarist Russia—prostitution and alcoholism—received diligent attention from the earliest days of Soviet medicine. Within a period of a very few years drunkenness was greatly reduced and prostitution was almost abolished. Practical measures were instituted in bringing these changes about—practical measures and common sense. Venereological institutes were established for the care and treatment of prostitutes. At the same time, they were also taught useful trades such as cooking, designing, dressmaking and weaving. They were taught the dignity of honest labor. Their economic status was improved. The only prostitutes who did not benefit from these procedures were the psychopathic personalities who required psychiatric treatment and isolation. This was given them, and the rate of venereal diseases dropped to an encouragingly low level.

Similar methods were employed in regard to chronic drunkards. They were deprived of their wages upon repeating their offenses. They were also educated along social lines and given some measure of respect for themselves and their families. Where required, medical and psychiatric care was made available to overcome the intense craving for alcohol.

Other social aspects of medical practice were attempts to eliminate maladjustment, emotional immaturity, and other failings among certain individuals in the society. Practical psychiatry did a great deal to ferret out hidden conflicts, bring them to the surface and institute corrective measures. Quirks in human nature, curious twists of the human mind, deviations from normal thinking and behavior received careful attention, and corrective measures were taken at once to overcome them. Thus, psychiatry served and continues to serve a very useful function in preventing the onset of more serious mental ailments and maladjustments.

From its inception, Soviet medicine was vitally interested in the economic status of the physician. As soon as the system of government medicine was adopted, it was made clear that the physician would be paid by the state and it was constantly emphasized that it was the doctor's duty to keep his patients well, no matter the cost, so that the services of no citizen should be lost in building up the new republics. It should be stated, however, that not all physicians worked for the state alone. There were a few exceptions. But all hospitals, sanitariums, clinics and dispensaries were and are state controlled and operated.

This does not mean that private medical practice is not permitted under certain conditions. For instance, a physician who has attained a great reputation in his specialty and whose skill is unique may be called in to give an opinion or to render special treatment, for which he may receive a fee from the patient in addition to his salary which is being paid him by the state. Dr. Kaminsky, the second Commissar of Health, encouraged private practice. He found that there was no conflict between private practice and socialized medicine. There need never be in any enlightened state. Under government medicine, as in private practice, certain physicians attain renown because of unusual skills and their services are not restricted. In the Soviet Union today, any physician may be called on to render his services to a private patient and be paid by that patient. No objection is ever raised by the state authorities. As a matter of fact, it is a rather common practice.

Dr. Frankwood Williams, who was very much interested in Soviet medicine which he studied at close range, said: "Crime, with all that we have done, is a serious major problem; nervous and mental diseases take their annual ghastly toll; maladjusted school children and adolescents continue to be a problem of great concern. In Russia, believe it or not, these things have ceased to be major social problems, or are rapidly diminishing as such. It is inconceivable, but there it is. The rate of incidence of nervous and mental diseases has risen in our country every year since statistics have been kept and the work of some of us who have been laboring in the field of mental hygiene for the past twenty years has not changed one-tenth of one per cent. And yet in Russia there is reason to believe that the rate of incidence of nervous and mental diseases is dropping.

"Has this been accomplished by some legerdemain? Is it by some trick that delinquency is not a serious major social problem; that alcoholism is steadily decreasing in social significance; that nervous and mental diseases are dropping not only surprisingly but unbelievably; that there aren't so many maladjusted school children; that adolescence in Russia is not a serious problem? This has not been accomplished by a trick that we cannot learn and apply here.

"Can Russia teach us? If we attempt to learn from Russia, it will be the hardest lesson we have ever attempted. And yet it is simple. What is it? Not tricks of education, not special methods of handling delinquents or nervous and mental conditions. It is merely this: that a civilization cannot be based upon the principles of exploitation, but that a civilization *can* be based on the principles of no exploitation. Everything else, education and all, follows from this."

Dr. Williams is apparently correct. The incidence of psychoneurosis among soldiers in the Soviet armies was less than in all other armies. There were very few mental breakdowns. Even the civilian population, subjected as it was to the horrors of war, still maintained a reasonable level of mental health. A satisfied and secure people is a mentally vigorous and healthy people.

The great Russian physiologist, Ivan Pavlov, said: "Science is now honored by the broad masses of the people in our country. . . . Science in former days was separated from life and was alien to the population. Now I can see science is esteemed and appreciated by the entire nation. I raise my glass to the only government in the world which could have brought this to pass, which values science so highly and supports it so actively—to the government of my country."

This statement is even more true today than it was in Pavlov's time. Interest in science is so widespread that the researches of the scientists are extensively reported in the daily press. Special movies of Soviet scientific accomplishments are shown in the theaters. Doctors and scientists who have attained special eminence are honored by the state with titles of "Academician," or even "Hero."

As we have seen in this chapter, the beginnings of Soviet medicine were brave beginnings. They foretold of much greater things that were to come. A veritable revolution took place in medical education, practice and research, a revolution that startled and amazed the rest of the world. From these beginnings stemmed many great discoveries and innovations in all branches of medicine. In subsequent chapters we shall examine these discoveries and innovations in greater detail.

II

MEDICAL EDUCATION

THE Soviet Union is the only country in the world which has undergone profound and revolutionary changes in the education of physicians within recent times. According to Dr. Michael B. Shimkin, the history of medical education in the U.S.S.R. falls into three general periods: reconstruction, experimentation and stabilization. From 1917 to 1922 the after-effects of the war and revolution were still very much in evidence. Conditions were chaotic; famine and epidemics were widespread and the medical profession which was essentially a holdover from the Czarist days was wholly inadequate to cope with them. The curriculum, which was modeled after the German, consisted of five years of didactic demonstrations, lectures and very little clinical application. Admission to medical school in the Czarist period was restricted to the privileged few. Sex, race and religion were determining factors. As soon as the Soviets came into power these restrictions were abolished. The pendulum swung in the opposite direction. Preference was given to the children of workers and peasants. Consequently, many students were not prepared to undertake the study of medicine, equipment was poor and there was a shortage of instructors. Examinations were a mere formality and many very poor physicians were launched on their careers. Medical training was at a low ebb.

After 1922 and up to 1930 there was a slow but decided improvement in the quality of medical education. Equipment was better; the number of medical schools increased.

Examinations were resumed and the students were better prepared to take them. Hygiene and preventive medicine came to the fore and these subjects were stressed in all medical schools.

In 1930 the First Five Year Plan was put into effect and medical education in the U.S.S.R. underwent a radical change for the better. The Commissariat of Public Health assumed the jurisdiction of medical schools from the Commissariat of Education. Physicians now had complete control of medical education, and the course of study was reduced from five to four years. The number of subjects was cut down, the use of outmoded Latin was abandoned, duplication was done away with, theoretical consideration was greatly reduced and practical clinical work was stressed. The social sciences found a place in the new curriculum; physical culture and military training assumed a very important role. Students worked in groups and examinations were again abolished.

Because of the peculiar problems of the Soviet Union, it became apparent that a greater emphasis on medical specialties was needed. Specialists were required for industries, collective farms, maternity homes, and health centers as well as for the usual clinical subjects. For this reason three faculties of medicine were established: general medicine and prophylaxis, hygiene and sanitation, and pediatrics—maternity care and child protection. As was to be expected three-fourths of the students took the general course. Ten per cent of the students were enrolled in the faculty of hygiene and sanitation.

Within a few years it was quite evident that the results obtained from this new medical curriculum were not satisfactory. First, there was a dearth of preclinical subjects which was later felt when the students undertook the clinical studies; many of them felt themselves to be poorly prepared. Second, there was too much overemphasis on non-therapeutic subjects. For these reasons revisions in the medical curriculum were again begun.

By 1935 the medical course was once more lengthened to five years; group projects and studies were reduced, more lectures and recitations were given, and Latin was resumed for medical terms. Also, examinations were resumed. At the same time, the quality and number of medical instructors increased, equipment was improved and the type of medical practitioner graduated from the medical schools was more sure of himself and better prepared to practice his profession.

In 1913, under Czarist rule, there were but 19,785 physicians in Russia; there were only thirteen medical schools with 8,600 students. By 1941 there were 130,348 physicians in Russia and 51 medical schools with 105,000 students. Great difficulties were experienced in the early years of the Soviet Union but medical education and care always received prime consideration. Medical education was continued without interruption during all national disasters, including war.

All medical affairs in the U.S.S.R. are under the administration of the People's Commissariat of Public Health; this includes medical education as well as allied professions, such as the training of dentists, pharmacists and other medical personnel—nurses and *feldshars* (medical attendants with training approximating that of a male nurse). The Commissariat has six principal divisions, including one on medical research and education. Under this division is a department of medical-educational institutions. Matters of policy and the more important questions regarding education are also considered by the Committee of Higher Education of the Council of People's Commissars of the U.S.S.R.

The Commissariat of Public Health of the U.S.S.R. actually has direct supervision over very few of the medical schools. Most of them are under the control of the Commissariats of Public Health of the constituent republics of the Soviet

Union. In 1941 there were some 72 medical institutes in the U.S.S.R., including dental, pharmaceutical and other closely allied colleges. In addition, there is a specialized medical school, the Medico-Military Institute in Moscow, which gives a complete medical course with emphasis on military medicine. This school is administered by military authorities. It is somewhat similar to our own Army Medical School in Washington, D. C., with the exception that the American school, also run by the army, is for postgraduate studies only, and admits only physicians who have been graduated from other medical schools and who have been commissioned in the United States army.

The various republics constituting the U.S.S.R. are all vitally concerned with medical education. There is at least one medical school in each of these republics. Naturally, attempts have been made to distribute the medical schools geographically and according to population.

In 1941 there were about 105,000 medical students in the U.S.S.R. As is to be expected the largest schools are located in the cities with the greatest concentration of population, namely, Moscow, Kiev, Leningrad and Kharkov. These schools enrolled an average of 3,000 to 4,000 students. The smaller medical schools, located in smaller cities, numbered several hundred students per school. Methods of education were the same in both the large and small schools, and the quality of training was uniform.

Postgraduate medical education is also under the direction of the Commissariat of Public Health. There are now some eleven postgraduate medical schools and they are not connected with the undergraduate medical schools. They are separate institutions and their work consists exclusively in postgraduate training of physicians who desire to go in for research work or who desire training in some specialty.

Education in the U.S.S.R. is given free to all citizens. Formal education usually starts at the age of eight and in the lower school lasts seven years. Three additional years are given in the middle schools. These ten years of preliminary education are equivalent to the primary and high school education in the United States. In general, studies include physics, chemistry, biology, mathematics and one foreign language.

In the United States a premedical education is required before admission to a medical school. This is not the case in Russia. After completing what amounts to his high school education, a student who has an outstanding record may be admitted to any medical school in the Soviet Union without any examination. If, however, the record is below standard, examinations are required before admission to the medical school can be granted. This examination consists of oral tests in chemistry, physics and mathematics, and an oral and written examination in the Russian language. Examinations for admission to medical school may also be taken by nurses, midwives and *feldshars* who have completed the subprofessional courses and have practiced for at least three years.

All examinations for admission to the medical schools are uniform and are set by the Commissariat of Public Health. Race, color, creed and even Communist Party membership are not considered in the admission of medical students.

In general, the number of applications for admission to medical schools in the U.S.S.R. are twice the number of places available. The average age of students applying for admission is seventeen to twenty, much below that of students in the United States. A curious thing is that women students exceed those of men. In 1939 the number of women physicians in the Soviet Union was 61 per cent. At the present time more than 85 per cent of the physicians in the U.S.S.R. are women.

In Moscow, Leningrad and in other capitals of the Soviet republics, there is an annual tuition fee of 400 rubles, while in other cities the tuition is 300 rubles. However, it is retained only until the successful completion of the examinations. Outstanding students are given scholarships. All medical students in the U.S.S.R. have special privileges which do not exist in other countries. They may obtain purchases at reduced rates; theater tickets are also sold to them at special rates.

At the present time, the medical course is still five years. There are two semesters in each academic year. The winter session is from September 1 to January 23, and the summer session from February 6 to June 30. As in the United States, new classes are admitted once a year, in the fall. There are six hours of classroom work a week. Instruction is for eighteen weeks a semester, with two additional weeks for review and preparation for examinations.

Today the medical schools still offer three different types of courses. The most popular course is that in general medicine which is taken by the great majority of the students; the second is a course in pediatric medicine in which child care and care of expectant mothers is emphasized. The third type is that of hygiene and sanitation, which is roughly similar to American courses in public health. The difference is that while in the United States sanitation and hygiene is primarily a postgraduate course, in the Soviet Union it is an undergraduate course. Probably that is why they have more specialists in public health than we do. These three types of courses are not available in all the medical colleges.

Within recent years there has been a tendency for a reduction in the differences in the three different types of courses. All these courses are five years in length and for the first five semesters they are identical. During the last five semesters the hygiene and pediatrics courses contain additional courses relating to their respective fields. Thus, the pediatrics course contains subjects in infant nutrition, hygiene of mother and child, school hygiene, education and psychology. The course on hygiene is divided into the following additional subjects:

industrial hygiene, epidemiology, community hygiene, nutrition and school hygiene.

During the freshman year in the Russian medical school, with the exception of anatomy and histology, the subjects taught are those usually found in American premedical courses. For example, biology, chemistry, physics, economics, philosophy. The second year consists of instruction in biochemistry, physiology and bacteriology.

The final three years are devoted to purely medical subjects, and most of the time is spent in laboratories and hospitals. The subjects taught are pathology, pharmacology, internal medicine, surgery and physical diagnosis. At the conclusion of the sixth semester, clinical instruction is emphasized and the students are sent to the various district clinics and hospitals where they spend four weeks exclusively in clinical work.

At the end of the fourth year, there is an additional seven weeks devoted entirely to clinical work in the district clinics and hospitals. In the specialized courses of pediatrics and sanitation all the practical work is done in these respective fields. Obstetrics is included in all three courses.

At the end of every semester, two weeks are devoted to preparations for written and oral examinations which are rigorous and test the students' theoretic and practical knowledge. Practical work is emphasized throughout the semester. At the end of the fourth year the student must pass a comprehensive examination which includes internal medicine, surgery, obstetrics and gynecology, neurology, dermatology, venereal disease and public health administration. It has been estimated that approximately 10 per cent of the students fail the medical course.

Various electives are available for all students. For promising students opportunities are available in research, and encouragement is given to develop any special talents in this direction.

As in the United States all graduates of medical schools must pass an examination given by the government before they can be licensed to practice medicine. The subjects in which the examination is given are internal medicine, surgery, contagious diseases, pediatrics, obstetrics, gynecology, hygiene, anatomy, physiology and pathology.

Upon successful completion of the medical course and licensing, the graduates are given the title of *vrach* (physician). In addition, they are given commissions in the Red army or navy reserves (women as well as men).

One conspicuous difference between graduates of American medical schools and Soviet medical schools is that all new Soviet physicians appear before boards of the Commissariat of Public Health and, in the order of their academic standing, choose assignments from a list of available positions. About 90 per cent of the new doctors are sent to rural areas, where they are assigned to posts for one to three years. At the end of this period they may apply for another position or for further training.

The most brilliant of the medical graduates are encouraged to engage in postgraduate medical training. A postgraduate course of three years, which leads to the degree of Candidate of Medical Sciences, is given. They may specialize in either preclinical or clinical subjects. In preclinical subjects, such as physiology or bacteriology, these doctors receive fellowships to work in medical schools or research institutions. If a clinical subject is chosen, they may specialize in medicine, surgery, neurology, psychiatry or any other specialty they choose. Before entering into any specialty they must have had three years of rural general practice or service as a resident in a hospital.

The graduate student doctors, during their fellowship period, are known as aspirants. During this time they assist in research and teaching and conduct special research in which they are particularly interested. They must also acquire a working knowledge of a foreign language. At the end of his period of study the graduate student or aspirant submits an original thesis which he defends before a committee of professors who satisfy themselves as to the aspirant's qualifications and express their decision by secret ballot. The names of those who have successfully passed the course are then submitted for approval to the Commissariat of Public Health.

The highest medical degree in the Soviet Union is that of Doctor of Medical Sciences (a degree which is also given in some postgraduate medical schools in the United States to graduate physicians upon completion of their courses). This degree is obtained after postgraduate work of at least three years—after acquisition of the Candidate degree. In order to obtain this degree the student must publish an extensive, original thesis approved by the entire medical faculty. This degree is not conferred by the medical school but by the Committee on Higher Education of the Council of People's Commissars.

Another very welcome innovation in Soviet medical education is that every doctor in the Soviet Union is required to take from three to six months of postgraduate instruction every three years. There are eleven postgraduate medical schools exclusively set aside for this work. During the time the physicians are taking this postgraduate course they are paid their regular salary and, in addition, are given an extra allowance to take care of expenses.

The faculty of the undergraduate and graduate medical schools is selected with great care. The deans are chosen from among physicians of professorial rank by the Committee on Higher Education of the Council of People's Commissars and the Commissariat of Public Health. The appointment is not for any fixed period. Each dean has one or more assistant deans who help him in the administration of the school. All policies are set by the heads of departments and submitted for approval to the dean and, if necessary, to the Commissariat of Public Health.

The faculty of the medical schools is selected from among physicians who have attained the degree of Doctor of Medical Sciences. All vacancies are given publicity in the newspapers and announcements are posted in the medical schools and other places. Qualified doctors are examined by at least three professors selected by the dean of the medical school from his faculty. The successful candidate is then appointed to his post by the Commissariat of Public Health. The newly appointed professor holds his position indefinitely and cannot be removed by the dean or by the Commissariat except for very extraordinary reasons.

Teaching is but one function of every department of the medical faculty. Productive scholarship is insisted upon. Research must be conducted and papers published on the results. This research work is closely supervised and evaluated by the professors of the school and submitted for approval by the dean to the Medical Research Council of the Commissariat of Public Health.

Department heads are mainly concerned with research and administrative work and do very little lecturing, four hours per week being the most usually devoted to lectures. The professors do most of the lecturing assisted by their *docents*. *Docents* are highly qualified, having earned the degree of Physician or of Candidate of Medical Sciences to be eligible. They deliver lectures on subjects assigned by the professor and otherwise assist in teaching and research.

Aiding the *docents* are assistants who usually already have the Candidate degree. They are also selected by the professors from physicians who are currently engaged in working for a higher degree. There is usually one assistant for every twelve students in the clinical subjects and one assistant for every twenty-five students in the preclinical subjects.

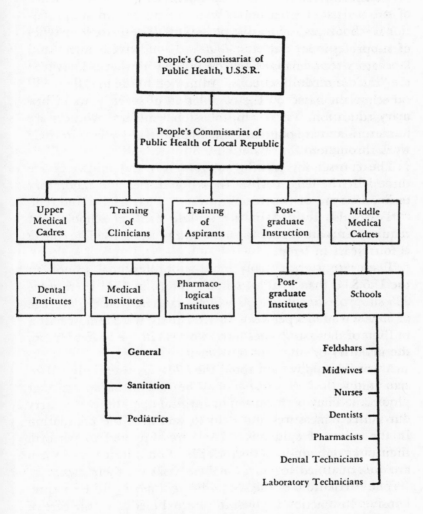

ORGANIZATION OF MEDICAL EDUCATION IN THE U.S.S.R.

A medical phenomenon in the Soviet Union is the presence of subprofessional personnel who are trained in subprofessional schools and who assist physicians. There are four types of subprofessional workers: *feldshars,* midwives, nurses and laboratory technicians. They are trained in what is known as the "middle medical schools." Admission to the middle medical schools is based on the completion of seven years of primary education. These subprofessional medical workers are numerous and are of great value in aiding physicians in their work throughout the Soviet Union.

The courses for training of *feldshars* and midwives are three years in length while those for nurses and laboratory technicians are of two years' duration. Pharmacists and dentists are also trained in the middle medical schools, but requirements are higher for these two professions. The course is four years in length.

There are a great many more subprofessional schools in the U.S.S.R. than medical schools. Thus, in 1941 there were 985 subprofessional schools which graduated on the average of 85,000 students per year. In 1941 there were almost half a million of these subprofessional workers in the Soviet Union, the majority of whom were women.

A word should be said about the *feldshar,* essentially a Russian innovation. A *feldshar* may be said to be an assistant physician. They perform minor surgical operations and carry out sanitary measures and help to vaccinate the population in the event of epidemics. They are supposed to perform their tasks only under a doctor's direction, but many of them are well-qualified to perform these tasks on their own.

The curriculum of the school for *feldshar* is quite comprehensive. Instruction is given in internal medicine, the care of patients, medical techniques, materia medica, infectious diseases, disinfection and inoculation, minor surgery and military science and tactics.

Midwives are also quite plentiful in the U.S.S.R. since the

great development of maternity homes and natal care programs. Midwives act as assistants to physicians in the maternity homes located in rural districts. They are qualified to perform a delivery when a physician is not present or available.

The nursing profession is not as highly developed in the Soviet Union as it is in the United States. Nurses are trained for two years, following which they become either medical nurses for duty in hospitals and clinics, or nursery specialists for the care of children.

Another point of difference between American and Soviet medical training is that no provision is made in Russia for an interne year. Upon their graduation, only the best students may receive further training in hospitals, or enter research institutes. The better students are assigned to districts where they have to depend solely upon themselves. The graduates in the last quarter of the class are sent to work as assistants to experienced physicians.

III

MEDICAL CARE THROUGH INSTITUTIONS

THE burden of medical care in the Soviet Union falls on the polyclinics, district medical centers and other medical establishments of varying sizes. Thus, every Russian citizen has some assurance of a medical center or establishment from which he can obtain the best advice and treatment that modern medicine can give.

Prior to the Revolution there were some 1,230 dispensaries in Russia, mostly concentrated in the larger cities. The rural and outlying populations could not take advantage of these dispensaries. Following the Revolution, new medical centers were established and care was made available in districts and localities which had never seen dispensaries before. Throughout the years there was a steady increase in the number of these health centers until by 1941 there were 13,461 medical centers or establishments in the Soviet Union.

The People's Commissariat of Public Health is in charge of all medical affairs in the U.S.S.R. and is therefore in charge of the medical centers throughout the land. The Department of Urban Medical Centers and the Department of Hospitals for Rural Communities have charge of the various medical establishments.

These medical centers or establishments are of different sizes and have different names for each type. The largest type of medical center is called a polyclinic. The next largest is known as an ambulatorium. There is another type of medical establishment called a dispensary which is rather specialized in function. The polyclinics and ambulatoria are, for the

42

most part, located in residential districts and industrial plants. The dispensaries are located at strategic points and are basically specialized units for the treatment and prevention of various diseases like cancer, tuberculosis, goiter, skin and venereal diseases.

The smallest of these centers are medical stations. They are staffed by physicians, or *feldshars* and nurses. They exist mainly for the purpose of administering first aid and routine treatments of various kinds; these stations are, in fact, outposts of the larger polyclinics and ambulatoria. They are located strategically throughout the land for the prompt rendering of first aid and other routine treatments which are most commonly required.

Still another type of medical center is the specialized medical station. They may be either independent establishments or outposts of large dispensaries. They are established in various localities in accordance with the needs of these localities. Their work is specialized to a high degree. Thus, in towns of Central Asia where trachoma is prevalent, these specialized stations function specifically for the prevention and treatment of this extremely infectious eye ailment. In localities where worm diseases are particularly prevalent these stations render treatment mostly for these diseases.

There is still another type of medical establishment— emergency stations—which are located in the largest cities, to treat victims of accidents and so on. The entire medical set-up is extremely flexible and is established entirely in accordance with the needs of the various localities for medical treatment.

The polyclinic is the largest type of medical center and is prepared to care for all cases that do not require hospitalization. The size of the polyclinic varies in accordance with the district in which it is established. As an example, the United Polyclinic in Leningrad has sixteen departments, a medical staff of 233 physicians, 256 consultation rooms and a total staff of 800 people. It also has a staff of consultants consisting of specialists who are called in for difficult cases.

A typical polyclinic consists of three departments: the department of clinical diagnosis which includes x-ray and laboratory divisions; the specialized departments which consist of the malaria, eye, ear, nose and throat diseases; and corrective gymnastics, physical therapy and neuropsychiatry divisions. The main departments of the polyclinic consist of internal medicine, with at least six physicians; surgery, with at least four surgeons; obstetrics and gynecology, with not less than three doctors; tuberculosis with not less than three physicians; dermatology and venereology, with at least three physicians, and dentistry with not less than five dentists. This is a very complete, compact and efficiently functioning medical unit.

The ambulatorium is a smaller type of medical establishment. The physician who is at its head is responsible directly to the health authorities or to the institution of which the ambulatorium may be a part, such as a hospital or a polyclinic.

The total staff of the average ambulatorium is usually not more than fourteen. The ambulatorium serves about 10,000 people. If the population is smaller the medical staff is correspondingly reduced in size. The staff consists of general practitioners and specialists who see patients not only at the ambulatorium but also in their homes.

The main departments of an ambulatorium are internal medicine, surgery, obstetrics and gynecology, and dentistry. The auxiliary departments consist of physical therapy, special treatment, x-ray and laboratory diagnosis. If the patient requires treatment which is not available in the ambulatorium he is referred to the polyclinic.

All physicians who serve in the various medical centers are on a full-time basis and they are paid by the government for their services. All the work (both laboratory and clinical),

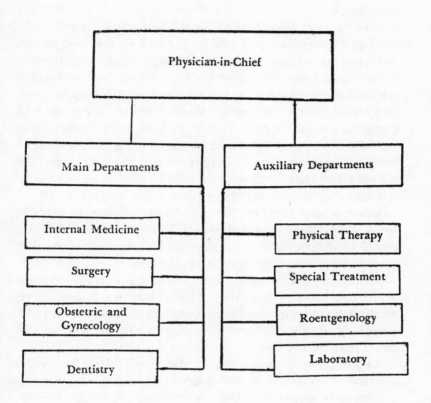

ORGANIZATION OF AN AMBULATORIUM

is carried out completely either at the medical center or at the patient's home. There is no charity medical work, subsequently all procedures are carried out carefully and to completion.

The medical centers, such as the polyclinic, the ambulatorium, the stations and others, are not merely out-patient departments as they are in the United States, run by physicians who give their services free. These are full-staffed medical units, run by doctors who are paid for their work, and consequently the best of medical service is rendered. A complete medical service is rendered not only in the center but also in the patient's home. An attempt is always made to see patients by appointment only, so that the best care could be rendered them unhurriedly.

Each medical center must know the people it serves, whether or not they are ill. Surveys are constantly made of housing and living conditions, studies are made of the incidence of disease, and measures are constantly instituted to prevent outbreaks of infectious diseases.

So health-conscious are the Russians that every district has a citizen's health committee. This committee has no direct administrative responsibilities, but it serves a very useful purpose by rendering aid and assistance to the medical workers in its particular district.

Another encouraging fact is that every block and every apartment house has its own health committee which is concerned with assisting in the operation of the medical center or unit which serves its district. As a matter of fact, it is part of the duty of the staff of the various medical units to organize such committees to render the medical work of these units more effective.

One of the prime functions of these block and apartment house health committees is to organize first-aid stations. The committee members are trained by the doctors from the local medical unit and they are prepared to render first aid at all times when medical aid is not immediately available.

One of the most important functions of the various medical centers or units in the U.S.S.R. is health education. Infectious diseases can be prevented in great part by education. The doctors of these various units give lectures, demonstrations, exhibits and discussions, and the people are taught about personal hygiene, child hygiene, the prevention of infectious diseases and accidents. Special courses are given which lead to the granting of Red Cross certificates. Health is emphasized as being of the greatest importance in any state or community.

One of the most important functions of the larger units like the ambulatoria is medical-prophylactic work which is done by a special member of the staff known as the visiting health officer, whose work consists mainly in examining and treating patients at their homes or places of business. He also supervises certain groups of patients. For example, a man who has had tuberculosis, has been to a sanatorium and returned with the disease arrested, needs constant supervision to prevent a recurrence. The visiting medical officer sees to it that this man leads a life consistent with good health.

Another important function of the visiting medical officer is the prevention of the spread of infectious diseases. If measles breaks out in a home, this doctor is on the spot, sends the patient to a hospital, disinfects the home, examines all contacts and treats them to prevent the spread of the disease.

Another function of the work of the visiting medical officer is sanitary prophylactic work. He makes surveys on the causes of illness and institutes measures to prevent the outbreak of these diseases. Preventive measures are instituted where possible to prevent the spread of any disease.

Through these various medical centers and units scattered throughout the length and breadth of the U.S.S.R. a permanent campaign in health education is constantly going on. For the most part this campaign has been successful as attested to by the decrease in the incidence of preventable diseases in the Soviet Union.

IV

THE ACCIDENT PREVENTION SERVICES

ONE of the phenomena of the Soviet Union was the rapid development of all industries. This immediately created another very serious problem for the medical authorities to consider, namely, that of accidents and accident prevention. Every type of industry has one or more industrial hazards. These hazards increase in direct proportion to the increased mechanization and development of technological processes.

In the early days of its organization, the Soviet Commissariat of Public Health undertook a survey of industrial accidents and their causes. It was ascertained that the primary causes of accidents in industry were: an insufficient number of protective measures and devices, the inexperience of the workers in handling more or less complicated machinery and carelessness.

It was the function of the Commissariat of Public Health to see that the number of accidents was reduced. First, various safety measures and devices were prepared and installed in the various factories throughout the land. The government released sufficient funds to each factory for the setting up of these safety measures.

The second step was in familiarizing the workers with the machines they handled. Courses were given to acquaint each worker thoroughly with the type of machine at which he worked. In addition, he was given courses in accident prevention and first aid in cases of burns, bruises, fainting, and so on. Also, posters were conspicuously displayed, explaining the protective devices on the machines.

This was but the beginning in the fight against accidents. Every local health department was charged with organizing first aid for their industrial workers. This was worked out along the following lines:

1. A network of first-aid stations was organized in each factory and industrial plant.

2. Physicians and nurses who expressed interest in industrial medicine were given courses of special training in this field, in addition to more general courses, such as hygiene and accident prevention. To augment the work of the doctors and nurses, men and women with special aptitudes were chosen from among the workers, and were trained in first aid.

3. Standardized methods for the treatment of various types of industrial accidents were established.

The following principles were adopted in the organization of the medical care of the injured:

1. First aid was always to be given at the place of the accident.

2. Surgical care and treatment was, if required, to be given later.

3. Specialized care and treatment was to be given wherever required until the patient was completely recovered.

As soon as an accident occurs, first aid is administered immediately by the worker himself, his neighboring worker, or by someone especially trained in first-aid work. Every department in the factory is supplied with a stretcher and a first-aid kit, completely stocked with all the necessary equipment and medicines. The industrial nurse in charge of the first-aid room is responsible for keeping this first-aid kit in order.

After first aid has been administered, the patient, if his injury so requires, is taken to the first-aid room. Factories in which the first-aid room serves less than one hundred workers have a trained nurse in charge; where more than one hundred workers are served, a physician is in charge.

The first-aid room is always open and staffed in case of accidents.

The nurse or doctor completes the first-aid treatment and then decides what future steps are to be taken. If the injury is slight the worker returns to his work. If it is severe and requires surgical treatment the patient is transferred to the traumatological clinic of the factory polyclinic. In the largest factories there are traumatological clinics in the factory itself. In the smaller factories all the severe cases are sent to the regional polyclinic which is organized for that purpose.

The traumatological clinic contains special operating rooms for disinfecting wounds, a dressing station, a room for fracture work, an x-ray department and a physiotherapy department. There are from five to ten beds for patients who require a temporary stay following operation. These clinics are open twenty-four hours a day, always ready to receive and treat patients.

The duties of the traumatological clinic are:

1. To diagnose the injury.

2. To treat the injury in the best way possible.

3. To decide what further treatment is required and to see that this treatment is given.

4. To determine the degree of loss of efficiency that the injury has produced.

All patients requiring ambulatory treatment receive it at the clinic. If the injury is of such severity as to require treatment in the hospital, he is sent to the hospital best equipped to give the particular treatment, i.e., surgical hospital, accident ward of a general hospital, special traumatological institute, and so on.

The traumatological clinic is chiefly concerned with treating the following types of injuries:

1. *Flesh wounds.* The wound is thoroughly cleansed with antiseptics and all foreign matter and dead tissue thoroughly removed. Then a few stitches are put in to bring the edges

together. In the great majority of the cases this is all the treatment required. The wound heals nicely in a short time.

2. *Dislocations.* Unless they are of an extreme nature all dislocations are treated at the clinic.

3. *Fractures.* Fractures of the fingers or the forearm are treated at the clinic. Fractures of the upper arm, the legs, etc., are treated at the hospital because hospitalization is required in these more severe types of fractures. In the cases of simple fracture the bone is set by hand; in the more complicated fractures special traction apparatus is used. In almost all cases plaster casts are applied.

4. *Bruises and sprains.* These are always treated at the clinic.

5. *Burns.* Simple burns are treated at the clinic. Severe burns in which extensive areas of skin have been destroyed are sent to the hospital for treatment.

6. *Occupational skin diseases.* Special attention is paid to occupational skin diseases, especially of those who work in chemical factories. A regular check-up is made of the hands of the workers in these factories and those showing chapped hands, cuts and bruises are sent to the clinic for treatment.

7. Patients suffering from injuries to the skull, spine, chest, abdomen, etc., are usually sent to the hospital for treatment.

Elaborate statistics and reports of the various types of accidents and where and how they occurred are kept at the traumatological clinic. These are studied from the point of view of increase or decrease in incidence, and where there is an increase steps are taken to decrease the accident rate.

Another function of the traumatological clinic is educational. Lectures are given at regular intervals on accident prevention. Moving pictures and exhibits are shown to drive home the value of safety in the prevention of accidents. The working public is thoroughly acquainted with protective and public health measures in industry.

At these clinics replacement examinations are also given.

All new workers are thoroughly examined from the point of view of suitability for the type of position for which they apply. They are then assigned to those departments for which they are physically best suited. Workers with physical handicaps accepted for a particular position are examined at regular intervals to ascertain the effects of the work on their condition. Also, workers with constitutional diseases, such as tuberculosis, anemia and metabolic disorders, are also examined periodically.

All polyclinics have assigned to them a number of beds in rest homes, convalescent homes, tuberculosis sanatoria, etc., for the factory workers under their supervision who may require such types of treatment. In addition, there is a staff of visiting nurses connected with each polyclinic who visit patients at their homes and give treatment and nursing care.

The traumatological institutes are specialized hospitals to which the traumatological clinics send the more severely injured patients. There are a number of these institutes scattered throughout the U.S.S.R., mostly in densely populated areas. There is at least one in each province and republic, more in the larger city areas. These institutes are staffed by surgeons who have received special training in the treatment of accident cases. All the latest apparatus is available and a blood bank is maintained in each clinic and ward ready for immediate use.

The object of these traumatological institutes is not only treatment of the more serious cases but also research in methods of treatment, and working out better and more efficient methods for the treatment of these cases. The chief institute for such study and research is the Central Institute of Traumatology and Orthopedics in Moscow.

After the patient has been completely rehabilitated he is returned to his factory. If there has been a loss of efficiency because of the accident a committee of medical experts determines the extent of this loss of efficiency and a new position which will not tax his strength is assigned to him. If, however, the worker is temporarily or permanently disabled he receives compensation. The case is then transferred to the Department of Social Security until such time as he is able to work again.

V

PUBLIC HEALTH

IN Czarist Russia public health was not only neglected, but there seems to be evidence that no obligation was felt on the part of the authorities to care for the health of the populace. The report of the Chief Medical Inspector of the Ministry of the Interior in 1913 is significant. In that year, ninety kopecks per capita were expended for public health, of which 94 per cent was for therapeutic aid and only six per cent for sanitary work including the struggle against epidemics. Russia at that time had the dubious distinction of leading all the European countries in the matter of mortality rate.

According to S. I. Mitskevich: "The peasant is not accustomed to and does not need scientific medical attention. His diseases are 'simple' and it is sufficient for him to be treated by a *feldshar*, while the doctor is only for the master class."

Organized medical care for factory workers and others was almost non-existent. Only 17 per cent of all factories and mills in Russia had their own hospitals. There were a great many factories which had no provisions for medical care whatsoever and resorted to private physicians only when it was absolutely necessary.

After the October Revolution, serious attempts to improve public health care and create a single governmental system of sanitary value were made. In the very midst of battle, the Revolutionary War Committee planned a medico-sanitary system which laid the foundations of the Soviet Public Health Department.

"As a basis for its activity in the matter of public health care, the Bolshevik Party proposes, first of all, the establishment of broad measures of sanitation, whose object will be the prevention of disease." With this declaration the need for a public health program was emphasized. The new government did not limit itself to the care of the sick. Prophylaxis on a nation-wide scale was instituted.

It was shortly after the Revolution that several governmental departments concentrated on questions of public health. In February, 1918, a medical council was created. This council unified the work of the various departments and on July 11th of that year the decree of the first Public Health Commissariat was published. The first problem was to control typhus which had spread alarmingly. Success was attained in arresting and controlling the typhus epidemic which at one time was so severe that Lenin said: "Either the louse will conquer Socialism, or Socialism will conquer the louse." Socialism evidently conquered the louse, which is the spreader of typhus.

During the First Five Year Plan, the Public Health Department extended prophylactic and therapeutic units of all types to cities and villages. There was a decided improvement in the quality of medical care. Clinics of various sorts and dispensaries were established in factories, which played a most important role in reducing the incidence of illness among workers as well as reducing industrial injuries.

Medical education was also reorganized. Specialists were trained in various aspects of hygiene—communal, industrial and nutritional. The quality of medical aid to maternity cases and children was vastly improved, with a corresponding reduction in mortality rates throughout the nation.

Hospital facilities for the population increased fivefold during the last twenty-five years. About three billion rubles have been expended for the construction and equipment of hospitals. By 1941 a half million beds were available in city hospitals. There was an improvement in the quality of institutional help, which was distributed more evenly and became accessible to all levels of the population. In 1941 there were some 35,000 physicians in the various city hospitals and more adequate care for the sick was provided throughout the country.

During recent years the U.S.S.R. built many sanatoria and health resorts, increasing the scope of public health work. In Czarist Russia health resort treatment was available only to the well-to-do. Now this type of treatment is available to the entire populace. These resorts and sanatoria have increased the number of beds to a total of half a million.

Clinics of various sorts have been established throughout Russia. In 1913 there were but 1,230 clinics and in 1941 there were more than 13,000. These are staffed by some 60,000 physicians. In these clinics are conducted extensive work in sanitary and public health education. As a result there has been an appreciable reduction in preventable diseases.

Industrial medicine has also advanced with giant strides in the U.S.S.R. Health measures have been introduced in all factories and mills. Constant supervision is maintained in all health measures, and as a result morbidity rates among workers in the largest enterprises of the Soviet Union has diminished.

As we have already seen, medical aid to the lower classes in Czarist Russia was deplorable. In all of Russia there were 4,142 township medical districts and about 5,000 *feldshars* (assigned to districts too small or poor for a physician), and about 49,000 hospital beds. The entire medical set-up for rural service in Russia in 1913 numbered about 6,500 physicians and 18,000 *feldshars.*

One of the first problems of the newly created Soviet Public Health Department consisted in rapid restoration and a considerable widening of health services for the peasantry and there was a steady growth in facilities for extending health and medical services to the rural districts. By 1941 there were more than 13,500 township health districts. The beds in rural hospitals, in comparison with the pre-Revolutionary period had increased three and a half times (175,000 beds) and the number of physicians four times (26,000 physicians).

At present, more than 70 per cent of the village soviets have a health center in charge of a physician health officer, assisted by a *feldshar* and midwife. In the Georgian and Turknebian Soviet Socialist Republics, all village soviets have medical facilities. During the war, all village medical centers were fully manned by physicians and middle-aged personnel. As a result of this thorough medical organization in the rural districts, the population of these areas is free of such epidemic diseases as smallpox, cholera and plague.

Care of women in matters of health was instituted shortly after the October Revolution. Specialized institutions were opened under the Soviet regime, and the Department of Public Health obtained sufficient sums necessary for the maintenance of mother and child care. During the past five years 200 new maternity hospitals were opened.

The development of nurseries in the Soviet Union is phenomenal. While in 1913 there were in the whole of Russia 550 cots in children's nurseries, in 1941 there were over 800,000 permanent berths and over 4,000,000 berths in nurseries which open in villages during the summer. There are now some 17,000 pediatricians and an additional 83,000 children's beds have been set aside.

In addition to the above medical facilities, special medical services are provided during the sowing and harvesting seasons to supplement the permanently established medical centers. Field services are set up to supervise the conditions of field work. Each traveling medical brigade consists of a physician, a *feldshar*, a nurse and a nurse's assistant. They supervise the meals, quality of the drinking water and other conditions which affect the health of the workers.

Another medical innovation of great importance to rural health in the U.S.S.R. is the traveling serological laboratory. Some 10,000 of these went to outlying districts in the U.S.S.R. in 1940 to combat infectious diseases. They accomplished a great deal in vaccinating 20 million of the populace against typhoid, 28 million against dysentery, 10 million children against diphtheria and 12 million against smallpox. Vaccination against smallpox, diphtheria and dysentery are compulsory in the Soviet Union and there is complete public co-operation in reducing the incidence of these diseases.

Within the past few years there has been a thorough reorganization of medical aid and health protection for the workers. Each large industrial enterprise in the U.S.S.R. with 250 or more workers has a health center on its premises at which workers and their families receive medical care. This health service functions on a twenty-four-hour basis and both the day and night shifts receive adequate medical attention.

Each of these industrial centers is manned by medical men who are thoroughly enthusiastic about their work. The medical director of the Tashkent Textile Combinat in the Uzbek Republic is but one example of many. In his region matters are organized on a thoroughly efficient basis. Doctors visit the shops at frequent intervals and give brief lectures on health matters. They go to the scene of an accident together with the trade union representative and sanitary inspector and make a thorough investigation of the circumstances contributing to the accident. Through such efforts, the Tashkent Textile Combinat has lowered the incidence of illness in the previous two years by about 40 per cent.

In addition to health centers in factories, mills and farms, there is a system of district health centers, and the citizen who is not already registered for medical service through his factory, receives medical care at his local health center. When he is too ill to visit the health center, he telephones for a doctor who visits him at his home. If his illness is serious enough to require hospitalization, his health chart is sent from the health center to the hospital, and, when his stay is over, this chart is returned to its point of origin. All such services are rendered without charge to the worker and his family.

Maternity care in the Soviet Union is highly and efficiently organized. Prenatal care is available to all women without charge. A woman gets thirty-five days leave of absence from work with full pay before the birth of her child and twenty-nine days of leave after that. Following this there is a provision for lighter work and no night work or overtime beginning in the fourth month of pregnancy. Because of this there has been a vast improvement in health among women and a reduction in the maternal mortality rate.

There is a slogan in the U.S.S.R. which says: "No Woman Must Give Birth to a Child at Home." In the five years following 1936 the number of maternity beds in the Soviet Union had more than doubled, increasing from 30,400 to 82,000 in cities and from 26,150 to 68,000 in rural areas.

There has also been an organized fight against abortions. Consequently there has been a rise in the birth rate, in spite of the fact that birth control information is readily available.

The science of nutrition has received wide recognition in the U.S.S.R. as a means of contributing to the public health. In 1941 a U.S.S.R. Vitamin Committee was organized by the health and food industry commissariats to plan and direct the theory and practice of food nutrition in the Soviet Union. One of the practical results achieved by this committee has been the establishment of special diet dining rooms in many factories to correct nutritional deficiencies of various sorts. Also prophylactic diets to decrease the incidence of occupational diseases have been worked out. Much information has come to light as the result of special nutritional research on the significance of vitamins in the prophylaxis and treatment of infectious diseases. The use of vitamins in the treatment of various nervous diseases has also received a great deal of attention. Vitaminology in relation to public health is receiving a great deal of emphasis.

Another very important public health institution is the Institute of Municipal Hygiene and Sanitation. This institute is concerned with many problems which have a close bearing on public health, such as removal of refuse, ventilation of dwellings, the odors and tastes of drinking water, suitability of clothing to climate, the health aspects of city planning, atmospheric pollution, and so on. Data gathered by this institute becomes the basis of public health regulations, such as dust, gas and smoke precautions to be taken by factories.

Because of the efficient work of the public health agencies, the leading killers—cholera, typhus and smallpox—have been practically eliminated. Even as far back as 1936 only 200 cases of smallpox were registered in the Soviet Union in the first six months of the year as compared to 2,827 cases in the United States. The six cases of diphtheria per 1,000 population was much lower than twenty per 1,000 in the United States. Typhus by 1936 had been reduced to a tenth of the figure of three years previously. In all other infectious and contagious diseases there have been notable reductions as the years went by. There has also been a notable decrease in occupational injuries.

At the head of the Public Health Commissariat is G. A. Miterev, who is a member of the highest administrative body of the Soviet Union, the Council of People's Commissars. He is assisted by two groups of experts: a Collegium, of which he is chairman, meets once a week to consider practical administrative matters and to draft orders and instructions which will be binding on all health institutions and workers; a Scientific Medical Council, consisting of over a hundred of the nation's leading physicians and surgeons, serves under Dr. Miterev and meets with him at stated intervals to consider medical problems. Under these men the public health of millions of people throughout the Union has improved considerably in the past few years.

During World War II the Soviet Public Health Department found its labors greatly increased. Dr. G. A. Miterev, its head, in an article *Public Health in the U.S.S.R.*, published in the August, 1945, issue of the *American Review of Soviet Medicine,* summarizes the accomplishments of his department as follows:

1. The Soviet Public Health Department studied epidemics and their causes arising in the course of the war. The first problem was the adoption of anti-epidemic and sanitary measures in the regions that were liberated from Nazi occupation.

2. Work continued on the following: (a) pathogenesis and treatment of war trauma, shock and reconstructive surgery; (b) the struggle against infections particularly among children; (c) nutrition and utilization of new nutritive resources in particular for children; (d) the development of theory and practice of anti-chemical defense and resources; (e) work on tuberculosis, cancer and arteriosclerosis.

3. New surgical methods were developed for the primary and secondary treatment of wounds. The Soviet Public Health Department adopted all advances in modern synthetic chemistry which enabled large-scale production of bactericidal and bacteriostatic compounds. The intensive study during the war of the microbic flora of wounds aided in the development of powerful specific biologicals for tetanus and other infections. Biologic and chemical preparations have been studied which stimulate rapid wound healing. The cytotoxic serum developed by Bogomolets is used in delayed union of bony fractures and chronic ulcerating wounds.

4. Intensive research is continuing for new treatment of

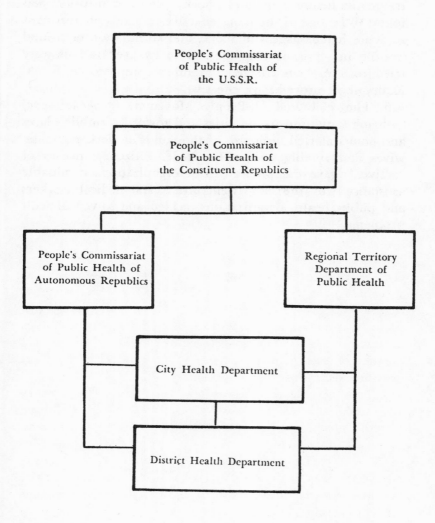

ADMINISTRATION OF PUBLIC HEALTH IN THE U.S.S.R.

traumatic hemorrhage and shock. Blood transfusion was found to be one of the more effective methods of treatment in acute hemorrhage and shock, and stimulation of wound healing in sepsis. During the war many preparations were tried to stop hemorrhage. Thrombin, prepared by V. A. Kudryashov, proved most effective.

5. The celebrated All-Peoples Movement (*geokchaiskoye*) to bring sanitation to the cities and towns, to public places and homes alerted hundreds of thousands of workers, housewives and intelligentsia. The Soviet citizenry, masses of "actives," gave the public health organizations invaluable assistance. For the past twenty-five years medical workers and public health organizations tackled and solved difficult problems.

VI

RURAL HEALTH SERVICES

IN spite of rapid industrial strides, the U.S.S.R. is still primarily a rural country, with 130 million out of a population of 190 million residing in rural areas.

The health of this vast population in the rural districts is of the greatest concern to the Soviets. In Czarist Russia the situation was badly mishandled. Thus, in 1913, there were but 4,367 medical stations, staffed with physicians serving the rural districts. In addition, there were 4,539 *feldshar* stations; rural hospitals contained 49,087 beds for general patients and 1,632 maternity beds. The medical set-up was wholly inadequate to care for a vast population of millions.

When the Soviets came to power they began almost at once to reorganize the medical services in the rural districts. This was done in an efficient and systematic manner. Each district in the Soviet Union has its own health department which has charge of all the medical services in the district. All these departments of health are responsible to a central department of health. Immediately, a Director of Rural Medical Services was appointed to the Health Department. Similarly, in the health departments which have rural districts under their jurisdiction, local directors of rural health services were appointed.

The most important medical institution that the rural health director controls is the medical center. This, in rural districts, combines hospital and ambulatorium. It has all necessary departments to render efficient medical services, such as medical, maternity, surgical, infectious diseases, x-ray, etc. The size of this medical center varies, of course, with the size of the community served. In general, an attempt is made to have five beds for every 1,000 population, and in many districts this goal has been attained.

A great deal of emphasis is placed in the U.S.S.R. on mother and child health, and for this reason special units have been established within the medical center. These are the Women's and Children's Consultation Center with gynecologists and pediatricians on the staff, and the other is the Maternity Home, staffed by obstetricians.

Each unit also has a completely staffed pharmacy which maintains a sufficient supply of all drugs likely to be used in the district. All the most recent drugs are stocked at all times and readily available to those who need them.

The rural medical center is always located at a point which is readily accessible to the farmers in the district it serves. In addition, there are medical stations located in the villages which are staffed by *feldshars,* nurses and midwives, who attend to the minor ailments of the rural populace.

Every collective farm, like every factory in the cities, has a health committee consisting of specially qualified medical workers elected by their fellow farmers. At regular intervals this committee meets to discuss the health problems of the farm, means of helping the health authorities improve health and sanitary conditions, training men and women for Red Cross activities, and so on. First aid is taught to all farmers so that they may be prepared to render first-aid treatment the moment it is required.

The Medical Director of Rural Health of each district has a disinfector on his staff, as well as a *feldshar* trained in the principles of sanitary engineering. This unit is sent to localities where there is a demand to improve sanitary conditions. Each such unit serves about 10,000 people.

As stated before, the maternity unit of the rural health department is regarded as of the greatest importance. Maternity care has been brought to the smallest villages and farms. The establishment of Collective Farm Maternity Homes in every rural community makes available the best of maternity care to every woman in all rural communities.

The average Collective Farm Maternity Home is of rather simple design and construction, consisting of four rooms— reception room, baths, delivery room and maternity room. It has from two to five beds, depending upon the size of the community it serves, and there is a midwife in constant attendance. A doctor can be reached at all times when his services are required. When a farm desires such a maternity home it contributes 75 per cent of the cost while the other 25 per cent is taken from the state budget.

The maternity service in the rural districts is well organized. When a farm woman becomes pregnant she goes to the Women's and Children's Consultation Center for examination. If a normal pregnancy is determined, she waits till labor pains begin, when she goes to the Maternity Home where her child is delivered in due course. She spends a week at the home, resting up and receiving instruction in the care and feeding of her child. If the pregnancy presents complications, the woman is hospitalized in the medical center where her case is handled by obstetricians who are prepared to handle any obstetrical difficulty and emergency.

After her discharge from the Maternity Home the woman returns at regular intervals to the Women's and Children's Consultation Center where her child is examined by the pediatrician and a record kept of its development.

In cases where the women are not able to care for their children because their services are required on the farm, the farm has a nursery which cares for the child while the mother is away at work. Now every farm and village has a nursery to take care of the children of farmers.

The rural doctor in the Soviet Union is at a much greater advantage than the rural doctor in the United States. The

Soviet doctor in the rural districts does not depend upon the farmers for his livelihood. He is paid by the state, and, being salaried, he is in much better economic circumstances than the American country doctor. His salary, as a matter of fact, is greater than that of a city doctor of like experience and occupying a similar position because his task is more difficult and his responsibilities greater than that of the city doctor.

The advantages of urban medicine have been brought to the country, and the presence of the rural medical centers with complete hospital and laboratory facilities permits the practice of scientific medicine which benefits equally both the doctor and farmer.

Another great difference between the American country doctor and the Soviet country doctor is that the latter receives one month's vacation every year with pay. After every three years of practice he receives a postgraduate course lasting at least three months, and during this time he receives not only his regular salary but a special allowance. Thus the country doctor constantly keeps up with the latest advances in medicine. Because of these provisions, he is a much better doctor and, best of all, the farmer receives just as good and just as scientific medical care as the city dweller.

In spite of its highly organized efficiency there are occasions when very special medical service is required which is not readily available in the rural districts, for example, brain or nerve surgery. It is quite obvious that the most highly trained neurosurgeons will be found in the cities with the greatest populations. Yet there are occasions when a farmer may have a brain tumor which requires treatment. For this reason, there is a very efficient coordination between urban and rural medical work. As an example, the Moscow District Clinical Institute has every type of highly skilled specialist on its staff. It serves not only the city of Moscow but also all the rural areas around Moscow.

Cases requiring the services of a highly skilled specialist

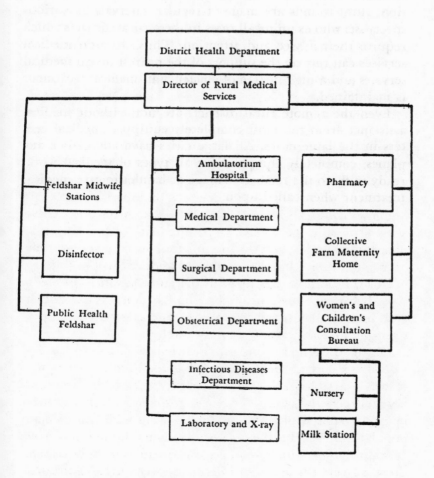

ORGANIZATION OF RURAL HEALTH SERVICES IN THE U.S.S.R.

from the outlying rural districts are referred to the urban district clinical institute where such cases are treated. In addition, rural rounds are made at regular intervals by various specialists who examine all cases in these rural districts which require their advice and attention. Thus all rural medical services can rely on the support of the nearest urban medical services and a high degree of efficiency in medical treatment is maintained.

Even the remote rural districts are not without medical assistance from the most completely equipped medical centers in the large cities. All large cities have ambulance airplanes, completely equipped for all types of medical work, ready to fly to the remotest village or hamlet to give medical treatment when called upon.

VII

HEALTH PROBLEMS CREATED BY WAR

DURING World War II many health problems arose which were handled with the utmost efficiency by the doctors of the U.S.S.R. Besides caring for the wounded, the spread of diseases, which is always accelerated during wartime, was prevented to a large degree. In former wars epidemics took more lives than bullets; this was not so true in the late world war.

From the very first days of the conflict the whole structure of health institutes and hospitals was united into one efficient unit for the prevention of disease. The public health service was under the direction of district physicians working in out-patient clinics in the cities and country. They came in daily, intimate contact with the vast population of the U.S.S.R.; they were the first line of defense in the war on infectious diseases. It was their duty to examine every person thoroughly for signs of disease, and every person with a contagious disease was hospitalized immediately to prevent its spread. This simple policy was extremely effective in preventing the spread of disease and the reduction in epidemics. During the war the number of hospital beds was increased 50 per cent to care for all infectious cases.

Of all the epidemic diseases there was an increase only in typhus. The typhus morbidity, having declined from year to year within the ten pre-war years in the Soviet Union had reached a low in 1940, when the disease occurred only sporadically. This decrease persisted until the last quarter of 1941. The greatest peak in the typhus epidemic was attained during the first quarter of 1942 which occurred in March. In April it began to subside again and during the winter of 1942-43 the incidence of typhus was half that of the corresponding period in 1941-42.

Another group of diseases which were found to have a tendency to increase during the war years were intestinal ailments, particularly typhoid and dysentery. In 1942 there was a moderate rise in the number of typhoid cases reported. Yet typhoid morbidity during the months of the second year of war was far below the incidence of the disease during many years of peace.

The public health officials remembered that cholera was a problem of vast importance in Russia during World War I, and for that reason measures were taken to prevent its occurrence in the Second World War. Large-scale vaccinations against this disease were carried out and careful check-ups were made. Thus far there has been no recurrence of cholera following the present world conflict.

Malaria is another disease intimately connected with war. In the United States we are painfully aware that malaria has increased tremendously. A great many thousands of our soldiers have been infected by it in various parts of the world. We now have many more malaria cases than we ever had before.

The same is true of malaria in the U.S.S.R. In 1941 the incidence of malaria rose considerably in several united republics such as Azerbaidzhan, Armenia, Uzbekistan and in numerous regions of R.S.F.S.R.—Gorkim Ryazan, Yaroslav, as well as in Dagestan A.S.S.R. In 1942 the average rise of malaria was only 0.3 per cent of the whole of the U.S.S.R. but there was a marked increase in twelve autonomous republics and in many regions of the R.S.F.S.R. as in Dagestan, Tambov, Chelyabinsk, Kuibyshev and Udmurt in the A.S.S.R. This increase persisted through nine months of 1943, and was due to the fact that during the confusion of war many prophylactic measures were neglected and drugs were not reaching these places when they should. In a short time these failures were corrected and the incidence of malaria began to decline.

Tuberculosis is another disease which flourishes in wartime. During World War I there was a considerable rise of tuberculosis in Russia. This was well remembered by the present health authorities. In order to enforce prophylactic measures against tuberculosis it was listed as an acutely infectious disease. Early segregation of tuberculous patients was practiced, timely and careful tracing of the contacts of all tuberculous patients were made and all persons with tuberculosis were immediately hospitalized.

Effective measures were constantly introduced to prevent the spread of the "white" plague. In January, 1943, the Public Health Council of the U.S.S.R. issued a special decree on methods to be employed in the fight against tuberculosis, and an active campaign was launched. All therapeutic, prophylactic and sanitary installations were mobilized. Hospital beds were increased. Immunization by the Calmette method was widely practiced. Educational propaganda was employed intensively.

Another problem which confronted the health authorities of the U.S.S.R. during the war years was the spread of venereal diseases. The Germans left behind them countless sources of infection in the areas temporarily occupied by them. This was confirmed by surveys made in the regions of Voroshilovgrad, Kharkov, Poltava in the Ukraine and in the regions of Kursk Stavropol and Krasnodar in the R.S.F.S.R. An active campaign to control the spread of venereal diseases in these sections was started soon after the Germans left.

It was noted that death from measles, whooping cough, scarlet fever and dysentery among children declined during wartime. At the same time an increase of mortality due to pneumonia and tuberculosis and a high death rate from diphtheria were noticed. According to Dr. G. A. Miterev the following conclusions are to be derived from these facts:

1. The trying evacuation period in the summer and fall of 1941, and in the fall of 1942, did not cause an increase of child mortality owing to a decline of infectious diseases.

2. The increased death rate from tuberculosis is a warning sign, necessitating a more energetic fight against childhood tuberculosis with large-scale employment of Calmette vaccinations.

3. The increase in the pneumonia death rate among children demands a change in the pediatrician's practice regarding hospitalization and therapy.

4. The central and local public health units are pledged to introduce all measures necessary to improve the health of the preschool and school child. The medical profession of the Soviet Union and the food administrations are coordinating their plans to secure better nutrition, vacations and recreation for all children who have suffered severely through the war.

During World War II a great deal was accomplished in matters of sanitation. Physicians, sanitary personnel and nurses cleaned out with their own hands the filthy houses left behind by the Germans, did all the necessary repair work and whitewashed the walls. From the first day of their arrival they gave medical care to the sick and wounded.

The greatest accomplishments were in the prevention of the outbreak of large-scale epidemics. The lessons learned in peacetime were applied with great effect during the war years.

VIII

CARE OF THE WAR WOUNDED

DURING the late World War Russia lost a great many lives and sustained many millions of war wounded. These wounded are now home, either in hospitals in the more severe cases, or receiving appropriate treatment at various out-patient departments and dispensaries.

Every wounded man and woman in the U.S.S.R. is guaranteed care and treatment. This is a fact which everyone in the Soviet Union understands because it is in the constitution of the U.S.S.R. The constitution grants every man, woman and child the inalienable right to security in old age and during illness or disability. This means that every wounded veteran has the right to be cared for, and more than that, his family also must be provided for.

According to law, veterans are divided into the following categories:

1. Totally disabled veterans who require hospitalization.

2. Totally disabled veterans who do not require hospitalization.

3. Veterans rendered unfit for their former occupations but capable of easier work with a shorter working day.

Pensions granted veterans vary according to rank. Each case is carefully studied by a Medical Labor Commission which consists of physicians and trade union specialists. Another factor taken into consideration when determining the amount of pension depends upon the type of disability and the veteran's former salary or wages. Thus, a private is granted a pension corresponding to 100 per cent of his average prewar earnings if he is totally disabled, and 75 to 50 per cent if he has been rendered unfit for his former occupation and is capable of easier work.

The scale for privates is not in excess of 400 rubles, but when average earnings were below 150 rubles, a pension of not less than 150 rubles is granted. For veterans who were neither factory nor office workers before enlistment a similar pension is granted. This group includes farmers whose cost of living is not quite as high as that of wage earners in the city. In general, non-commissioned officers receive pensions that are 25 per cent higher than those of privates. The People's Commissariat of Defense determines the pensions for commissioned officers, each case being considered on its individual merit. A veteran continues to receive his total allotment no matter how high his earnings are when he returns to work. For some rather strange reason, an exception is made in the case of farmers whose pensions are reduced 20 per cent.

The pension system is highly organized. Pensions are administered by the People's Commissariat of Public Security of the U.S.S.R. through departments in each republic. The Commissariat maintains offices in the territories, regions, districts and cities and are under the supervision of the local Soviets. At the same time the Commissariat of Social Security also maintains a network of medical institutes, polyclinics, laboratories, schools, rest homes, sanatoria and other institutions. It also has control over various cooperative organizations, such as invalids' cooperative societies.

The Social Security organization assumes care of the veteran before he has been discharged from the hospital. He is acquainted with his rights under the law. When he leaves the hospital a veteran receives his certificate of disability and his pension for a month in advance. After that he receives it from the local office, and when necessary the pension is delivered to his home. The Social Security organization also arranges pensions for those who are sent home directly from the front without having to go to a hospital. All pensions start from the day of discharge from military service.

The work of the People's Commissariat of Social Security is concerned not only with pensions for veterans but with the wider problems of rehabilitation of the war wounded, training them for new trades and professions if their disabilities render them unfit for their former work. The problem of rehabilitation is not merely limited to finding work to provide a meager subsistence. It is concerned with training the veteran to do useful and sometimes highly skilled work which results in good wages, interesting employment and easier working conditions.

The task of finding suitable work for veterans is solely that of the Social Security agencies. Plants and offices are constantly visited by Social Security workers who determine what positions can be filled by war veterans. The law stipulates that managers of factories, offices and public institutions must "in the shortest possible period of time and without delay provide suitable employment for invalids of the present war who have been sent to them by the Social Security agencies, approaching each case on its own merits and facts in assigning work." The law further states that adequate working and living conditions must be provided. These conditions are constantly checked by Social Security and trade union workers.

Retraining programs are begun in the hospitals. This is continued in the factories and offices, which furnish equipment, tools, raw materials and instructors. After their discharge from the hospital, the trainees are assured of employment in these plants.

The Social Security Commissariat also enters actively in the training program. It has established manual training shops and industrial and agricultural schools where short courses are given. For example, there are three large vocational schools for ex-service men in Moscow alone. Tuition is free and students receive stipends in addition to their pensions.

The Social Security Commissariat is also concerned with the problem of restorative medical treatment and prosthesis. In modern workshops under the supervision of the Social Security agencies, designers and medical specialists produce artificial limbs, orthopedic footwear, hearing devices and other aids. The cost of manufacture and fitting is borne entirely by the state. The local Social Security agencies certify the disabled needing artificial limbs. Traveling brigades of highly trained specialists fit veterans who live far from the workshops or factories.

Proper treatment and fitting of artificial aids reduce considerably the period of hospitalization and increase the patient's working ability. The Moscow Scientific Research Institute of Prosthetics, under the direction of the People's Commissariat of Social Security, has done great work in refitting the severely wounded veteran and restoring him to usefulness. The institute, which has its own hospital, has developed a method of early reamputation of the stump which considerably shortens the period of treatment. From two to four months after the first amputation, the patient is correctly fitted and is able to go back to work.

Another medical organization which is doing remarkable work in restoring the war wounded to a life of usefulness is the Central Institute of Medical Consultation and Rehabilitation of Veterans. It is now working on the problem of restoring motor function of injured limbs. Patients who have lost their legs are given special supports for standing and sitting. The institute has perfected a device which enables the severely crippled to work in the shoe industry. With the aid of another device one-armed men can stencil, while still another device enables the blind to work successfully at stamping various articles.

The program of rehabilitating the war wounded is not limited to pensions and allowances, medical care, help in returning to gainful employment and restoration of working ability. The state also grants the war injured a number of exemptions and privileges after he is employed. He receives an annual vacation and is not required to work overtime. If he is ill, the disabled veteran receives full pay regardless of the length of time he has been employed, while other workers must have been employed for a specified period of time before they are entitled to full sickness benefit.

Various tax exemptions are also granted. War wounded of the first and second categories pay only half the agricultural tax, and disabled collective farmers are exempt from deliveries of grain, rice and potatoes to the state. If there are no able-bodied members in the family, the ex-service man is completely exempt from the agricultural tax as well as from all deliveries in kind to the state.

The veteran receives all the medical aid he requires without cost to himself. He is entitled to the services of the most highly skilled specialists at all times. The Social Security agencies are pledged to care for him for the rest of his life, and they have been doing and are doing a magnificent job.

IX

THE CONTROL OF INFECTIOUS DISEASES

DURING twenty-five years that the Soviet Health Department has been functioning, many of the infectious diseases such as plague, cholera and smallpox have practically been eliminated. Others, such as the dread typhus and typhoid fever have been greatly reduced in incidence. This was brought about by a systematic study of the epidemic diseases in the U.S.S.R. and the taking of appropriate measures to bring them under control. The adoption of such measures as adequate prophylaxis, the reporting and hospitalization of all infectious diseases, disinfection of infected areas, education and early diagnosis of suspected cases has done much to control infectious diseases in all parts of the U.S.S.R.

Sanitation has become a highly respected science in the Soviet Union. Strict control is maintained over the water supply, the milk supply, food and other avenues through which epidemic diseases may be spread. Known carriers of typhoid and other infectious diseases are kept under special supervision and control.

Immunization and vaccination are now common in the U.S.S.R. Immunization of great numbers of the vast population has already been accomplished. In 1898, Dr. Visikovitch vaccinated 235 soldiers in a very timid gesture. In Czarist Russia vaccination was much frowned upon, and very little vaccination of the populace was done. The army was against vaccination as were many of the doctors. For that reason infectious diseases were widespread and in many districts rampant.

From the inception of the Red Army compulsory immunization was insisted upon. In 1919, the number immunized was 306.6 per 10,000 men; in 1920, 700.2; in 1921, 679.1 and in 1922, 999 per 10,000 men. In later years these proportions were increased considerably.

Thus, typhoid fever is practically non-existent. Regular immunization of the populace is insisted upon just as it is in the army.

Whenever there is a threatened outbreak of a disease, special immunization measures are instituted at once. The entire medical organization, from the local village doctor to the district doctor of the city clinics, is thrown into high gear to combat the threatened outbreak. Everybody is immunized against the disease and in 1938 the level of immunization among the urban population in the R.S.F.S.R. equaled 155.2 per 10,000 population.

Another disease of widespread occurrence in Russia, dysentery, now also is under control. Much pioneer work was done in investigating this vexing problem. Physicians throughout the Soviet Union set about investigating the epidemiologic peculiarities of dysentery in general and of its various manifestations in different parts of the country. Dysentery carriers were studied and put under control.

As a practical measure bacteriologists devoted themselves to a study of the different types of dysentery and prepared vaccines to control and combat this disease. Wide use has been made of the bacteriophage in the treatment of this disease, and good results were obtained in controlling several outbreaks.

Because children are particularly susceptible to intestinal diseases, particularly dysentery, special measures have been taken to organize hospitals and sanitary institutions for young children suffering from a chronic form of dysentery. Also, stations were established for those with acute intestinal diseases to expedite early diagnosis and prophylaxis.

Typhus was the big problem in Russia during the First World War. After the October Revolution a great deal was done in the fight against typhus. The entire medical organization was mobilized to combat it. The People's Commissariat of Health created a special anti-epidemic commission. Other commissions were set up in various areas and went into action against the epidemic.

In 1910 the Czarist Senate declared that it was not necessary for county hospitals to admit patients with communicable diseases when there were no wards for them. In contrast the Soviet health organization set aside hundreds of thousands of beds for infectious and contagious diseases. By the year 1920, 250,000 such beds were already available. Disinfecting stations were set up all over the country. Lectures were delivered on sanitary measures, posters were distributed as were booklets which taught the populace hygiene. Slogans were made popular, such as, "The fight for cleanliness is the fight against lice."

A great army was enlisted in the fight for cleanliness and the battle against the louse. Hundreds of thousands of workers were organized into groups for an active campaign against filth and disease. Various other measures were adopted such as CLEANLINESS WEEK, WEEK OF EDUCATION IN SANITATION and BATHING WEEK.

The central government alloted generous financial aid in this work. The entire medical profession was geared for quick action, as were hundreds of other organizations. The people joined in the fight—various committees were organized and much was done in the way of education along hygienic lines and all with very good results.

It is now clearly established that since 1921 the incidence and morbidity from spotted fever and recurrent typhus has shown a decided if gradual drop. From 1923 there has been a constant decline in the incidence of parasitic typhus.

Other diseases which have been put under control are the common diseases of childhood, particularly diphtheria. Wide hospitalization and early treatment at the first suspicion of diphtheria have brought about a decrease in the incidence of this disease which formerly was taking a heavy toll.

Immunization against diphtheria is now compulsory for all children between the ages of one and eight. The number of children immunized has been growing from year to year and, in 1940, 10,000,000 children were immunized against diphtheria. Reimmunization is also now commonly employed. Because of this there has been a sharp decline in the incidence of diphtheria. For example, in 1906 to 1910 it was 27.4 per 10,000 population, and in 1910 to 1913 it rose to 31.4, but in the early years of the republic, it began to decline, and in recent years it has never been higher than 7.6 per 10,000 population.

Russian bacteriologists are engaged in improving the quality of vaccines and other biological preparations so that more effective preparations may be prepared which would require less frequent injections and which would give protection against infectious diseases for much longer periods of time.

Another infectious disease which has held the attention of Soviet doctors is measles. The ability to reduce the incidence of this disease was limited because of an almost 100 per cent susceptibility to this infection and the lack of any specific immunization. In the early years of the Soviet Union the measures taken against this disease consisted of raising the resistance of the whole child-population, improving medical service to children and improving living and hygienic conditions in general.

In later years there developed the idea among Soviet physicians of producing a temporary immunization against measles. This method is now universally used by the various stations of the Soviet health departments throughout the country. Immunization of children first began in Moscow, Leningrad and other large cities, but it is now widespread throughout the entire republic.

The first such preparations consisted of a serum derived from the blood of convalescents, but now a serum prepared from adult's blood and a placental extract is used and it has been found to be very effective. In fact, so effective is this serum that there has been a great increase in the number of laboratories producing it.

The inoculations against measles as well as other prophylactic measures are carried out free of charge in all children's hospitals, child clinics, health stations, and so on. These inoculations are given to all children who have had contact with measles patients. The aim of prophlactic treatment is to raise the age of measles patients, to reduce the current incidence of the disease and to create an immunity by developing an abortive form.

Infectious diseases are now well under control in the U.S.S.R. Various prophylactic stations are established throughout the land to immunize the populace against all the common communicable diseases. Great progress has been made in reducing the incidence of all epidemic diseases.

X

THE WAR ON TUBERCULOSIS

IN spite of the fact that tuberculosis has always been endemic in Russia from the earliest times, very little was attempted by the Czarist regime in the way of curbing it. Toward the end of the rule of the Czars a single serious attempt was made to study tuberculosis at close range and to evolve means of caring for and treating tuberculous patients when the Pirogovsk Society organized the All-Russian League for the Struggle Against Tuberculosis. In 1912 the league had under its direction some forty-three dispensaries and eighteen sanatoria with 308 beds. However, with the onset of the First World War the number of these institutions was gradually reduced so that in 1917 there were only four dispensaries with 200 beds.

With the coming of the Soviet regime a systematic campaign against tuberculosis was organized with great effect. By 1920 a network of dispensaries and sanatoria was organized and staffed with specialists in tuberculosis. The sanatoria were located in those parts of the Soviet Union best suited by climate for the care and treatment of tuberculosis. All these institutes were organized and supported by the state. By 1921, 15,751 beds were available in 208 tuberculosis institutions in the R.S.F.S.R. and forty institutes with 3,640 beds in the Ukraine. By 1941 there were 1,048 anti-tuberculosis dispensaries and stations in the U.S.S.R. Also by 1941 there were 211 day and night sanatoria with 7,526 beds, of which 2,642 were for children.

The dispensary is the chief center in which all anti-tuberculosis work is initiated. Here is combined the prophylaxis and treatment of tuberculosis in its incipient stages. In the beginning of the campaign against tuberculosis tens of thousands of workers were examined for signs of the disease. A little later mass x-ray examinations of the chest were carried out and many cases of early and late tuberculosis were thus detected. Diet planning was inaugurated in special dining rooms in the large factories, for the care of early cases of tuberculosis. In 1935 in Moscow diet planning was made available to 1,735 tuberculosis patients. These special diets produced a very noticeable reduction of morbidity and a very significant rise in the working efficiency of those afflicted with tuberculosis.

Legislation by the various republics in the Soviet Union was enacted to protect the people against tuberculosis. Among other things this legislation provided for compulsory examination of all persons employed in the food industries and children's establishments, isolation of the tuberculous from workers' and students' dormitories, the compulsory notification of dispensaries concerning active cases, disinfection of homes of those afflicted with tuberculosis, and regulations regarding the use of milk from affected animals.

By far the most important function of the tuberculosis dispensary is prevention. Care of the sick in their own homes and the teaching of rules of hygiene by visiting nurses has acted in a very large measure to prevent the spread of infection.

Particular attention has always been paid to tuberculosis in children. Prevention of infection has, in this instance, been considered of the greatest importance. Medical and prophylactic care of tuberculous children are given by tuberculosis dispensaries, children's hospitals and sanatoria.

Among the most important duties of all doctors in the Soviet Union is the early diagnosis of tuberculosis in children. Examination of children's groups in nurseries, children's parks and summer playgrounds is carried out regularly.

In Czarist Russia the great majority of patients with tuberculosis of the bones were doomed to become crippled, because little was done to help them. In the Soviet Union today special attention is being paid to the early detection of bone tuberculosis and measures are instituted to prevent the spread of the disease; in this way crippling is minimized.

There are many physicians in the U.S.S.R. today whose specialty is that of tuberculosis. In 1919 intensive training of physicians in specialized fields was begun. By 1922 there were excellent specialized courses in tuberculosis conducted at Moscow, Leningrad, Krasnodar, Yalta, Kharkov, Kiev, Odessa and Kazan. Since 1932 the Central Tuberculosis Institute has conducted a corresponding course for rural doctors.

Within recent years the campaign against tuberculosis has been intensified. For the broader conduct of anti-tuberculosis measures more active utilization of the general public health network, the district doctors, pediatricians, therapists, sanatoria doctors and state inspectors were initiated.

An edict by G. A. Miterev, the People's Commissar of Public Health, brought about more concrete methods for fighting tuberculosis. District doctors were instructed to conduct public health work in the tuberculous homes in their own districts. The sanatorium epidemiologic dispensaries were instructed to carry out complete disinfection in the homes of all registered active cases. The state inspectors were charged with the responsibility of permitting patients with active tuberculosis to work in children's institutions, schools and food industries.

For the hospitalization of tuberculous patients from densely populated quarters, tuberculosis branches in local hospitals were opened. Also opened were special hospital beds as needed at the expense of the epidemiologic fund. During the year 1942, 5,000 additional beds were provided. Also opened were day and night sanatoria, special dining rooms in factories and tuberculosis dispensaries for adults and children.

Anti-tuberculosis measures reached their highest level in 1934 after the institution of the Council of People's Commissars on May 1st. This organization directed that there be developed an additional 12,000 hospital beds. 7,000 beds in night sanatoria for workers, 3,000 beds in day and night sanatoria in tuberculosis dispensaries, 15,000 places in children's gardens, summer schools for 6,000 children and invalid homes of 3,000 beds. Also, the Council of People's Commissars created funds for the increased nutrition of 100,000 tuberculosis workers in the defense industries and organized instruction for the All-Union Central Council of Trade Unions and for the Narkomzdrav of the U.S.S.R. concerning the arrangement of labor for those sick with tuberculosis.

The decree of the Council of People's Commissars has been carried out with great success by all the branches of the U.S.S.R. The Narkomzdrav of the U.S.S.R. has been aided by the People's Commissariats of the All-Union Central Council of Trade Unions in the development of anti-tuberculosis measures. Much has been accomplished in the way of halting the spread of tuberculosis in the Soviet Union.

XI

THE CONTROL OF MALARIA

IMMEDIATELY following the First World War there was a malaria epidemic which raged over most of Europe. Russia was one of the worst sufferers from this malarial scourge. Among the first duties of the new Russian government was to set up anti-malaria stations to combat the outbreak. In 1920 the Tropical Institute was established in Moscow. From the very beginning this institute became a center for research in malaria, and here plans were formulated for the establishment of branch anti-malaria stations, clinics and institutes throughout the Soviet Union. Physicians were trained here in anti-malarial work and dispatched throughout Russia to aid in the fight for freedom from this scourge. From this first anti-malarial institute in Moscow was evolved the present Martsinovsky Central Institute for the Study of Malaria and Medical Parasitology, one of the most famous institutes of this kind in the world today.

At the present time the war on malaria is highly organized in the U.S.S.R. There are at least eight institutes devoted exclusively to the study of malaria and medical parasitology. In addition there are a number of central malaria stations located in the capitals of the U.S.S.R. and autonomous republics. This work in malarial control, treatment and prophylaxis is carried out by 1,200 urban and rural malaria stations and 1,500 special clinics where patients may obtain medical treatment. In addition to these special anti-malarial organizations, the various anti-epidemic stations and rural health centers, whose work is concerned mainly with infectious diseases, also does anti-malarial work. Together these two types of organizations maintain a rather complete control over the malaria problem in the U.S.S.R.

Physicians whose work takes them to malarial districts are assisted by a highly organized group. These groups are made up usually of an anti-malaria brigade consisting of three persons, two of whom are engaged in prophylactic work and the third in treatment. There are some 4,000 such brigades in the Soviet Union. In addition similar brigades are trained on collective farms, in industrial plants, and timber and peat cutting camps for the purpose of carrying on effective antimalarial work, which is done under the control and supervision of the local medical authorities. It is estimated that there are 50,000 people working in these brigades and these are maintained by the farm or industrial organizations concerned. Their training is received at the district or urban malaria stations.

The central government in the U.S.S.R. maintains strict control of the malaria problem through the People's Commissariat of Health, which has a special department devoted exclusively to malaria. Similar malaria departments are maintained in the various other departments of health situated throughout the Soviet Union. Every year in the main department of health a plan for anti-malarial work, which provides for measures of control, prophylaxis and treatment is drawn up. In effect this plan is based on epidemiologic data. It is made up of three sections: (1) measures for eliminating sources of infection, (2) measures for destroying the anopheles mosquito which spreads the disease, and (3) prophylactic measures to prevent infection and the spread of infection.

A new departure in the control of malaria in the Soviet Union is the registration of all malaria patients, which is compulsory. It is a well-known fact that the malaria patient is himself a very potent source for the spread of malaria, because he retains the malarial parasites in his blood for a great many years. Periodic examinations are made of the entire populace in all malarial districts. Winter is the time selected for these examinations which are thorough and in which special records are made of all new cases and recurrences of old cases. Special treatment is given to all those who have had malaria during the previous year, in order to prevent a recurrence. Soviet malariologists have demonstrated that a month's course of treatment in April or May, depending on the season in which the greatest number of relapses is reported, has the effect of decreasing the number of recurrences to one-third or one-quarter of that observed among patients who are not given this treatment. Because of this the spring treatment of malaria patients is compulsory in the Soviet Union.

The method of treating malaria in the U.S.S.R. is that generally accepted throughout the medical world. This consists of a month's treatment with atabrine, given in three cycles. The first of these cycles consists of 0.3 gram a day for five successive days; this acts in controlling the acute and very distressing symptoms. After an elapse of ten days the same dose is repeated for three days and is repeated again after another ten day interval has elapsed. The purpose of the second and third cycles is to prevent early recurrences. This method has been tested on a great number of patients suffering from various types of malaria under different climatic and geographic conditions. It has been demonstrated that the application of this method completely cures 60 per cent of the patients.

It is well known that atabrine has very little effect on the sexual forms of the malarial parasite. For this reason all malaria patients and carriers are treated with atabrine in combination with 0.02 gram of plasmochin, a quinodine preparation which effectively attacks the sexual forms of malaria parasites. If the first attack of malaria occurs during the first half of the year these patients receive a second course of treatment in the autumn. The course is identical except that the dose of atabrine is reduced to 0.2 gram daily.

During the years 1942 and 1943 research workers at the central anti-malarial institute worked out two new modifications of the method of controlling malarial attacks. The first modification consists of giving the patient 0.5 gram in two doses of atabrine on the first day followed by 0.3 gram daily for three days, so that the first cycle is reduced to four days. According to the second modification, the patient receives an intramuscular injection of 6 c.c. of 5 per cent atabrine and 1.3 grams by mouth on the first day of treatment and 0.3 gram on the second and third days. Because of this the cycle is reduced to three days. The two other three-day cycles follow the original method with an interval of ten days between them.

Widespread and mass epidemiological chemical prophylaxis is regarded as of the greatest importance in the U.S.S.R. Preventative measures are carried out in regions of the vast land where it is impossible or economically impracticable to eliminate the malaria-carrying mosquito. Such places include fishing grounds, rice fields and small settlements in swampy districts. As a general thing, the measures taken to annihilate the mosquitoes do not destroy them completely in such places and those that remain are sufficient, particularly where malaria patients exist, to maintain conditions favorable to the spread of malaria. It has been found that under these circumstances it is more practical to devote all the attention to the patients as a source of the spread of infection.

The prophylactic method employed consists of the following: every person infected with malaria the previous year is rightfully regarded as a potential source of infection to mosquitoes throughout the malaria season, which is from April to May, and from September to October, and for this reason he receives two to three tablets containing 0.1 gram atabrine and 0.02 gram plasmochin for two days each week.

This method has been shown to result in a decided decrease in the number of fresh cases even in areas where there are great numbers of mosquitoes.

The second part of the anti-malarial campaign consists of measures directed against the mosquito itself. The first act consists in the destruction of the larvae of malaria-bearing mosquitoes in swampy districts. These measures consist of sprinkling Paris green from airplanes in swampy districts around large cities situated on the banks of wide rivers, like the Kuibyshev, Kazan, Rostov, Saratov, Astrakhan, Voronezh and others, at peat workings, and in rice fields. Before World War II five to eight million acres of anopheles-bearing water deposits were sprayed in this manner. The larvae are also destroyed on the ground by a special type of motor spray invented in the Central Institute and by various manual methods. Spraying of water deposits with a kerosene suspension of Paris green is the method widely used in the U.S.S.R.

Another means of combating malaria is the *Gambusia affinis,* imported from Central America and bred in the Transcaucasian and Central Asiatic Republics. Special reservoirs have been constructed to breed this fish, and in the spring the fish are distributed among the rivers, lakes, swamps and paddy fields.

Special funds are allocated among various bodies to fight malaria in the U.S.S.R. Special research is going on all the time to kill the larvae of the malaria-spreading mosquitoes. Preparations made from pyrethrum and other insecticides are employed with great effect.

In addition widespread education among housewives, school children, factory workers and others have brought home the danger from the malaria-spreading mosquito and various campaigns for the destruction of this pest have been organized with very good effect.

The third part of the anti-malaria prophylactic plan concerns the protection of healthy people from malaria infections. Information on means of protecting oneself against this pest has been widely disseminated. Windows are covered with metal or cotton gauze and people are provided with netting. Metal and cotton window screens are provided free of charge.

A great many substances have been tried which repel mosquitoes when sprinkled on the skin or clothing. Unfortunately, most have proved unsuccessful. Anabasine sulphate, which is widely used as an insecticide against farm pests proved efficacious against mosquito bites. Although the solution does not keep the mosquito away entirely, the number of bites are reduced considerably.

Within the past few years the malaria menace, instead of decreasing in the U.S.S.R., has increased. This is due to the fact that the German occupation has greatly increased the number of malaria cases. The network of anti-malarial stations in the eastern part of the Ukraine and the north Caucasus were completely destroyed during the German invasion. However, work of reconstruction has already begun.

Anti-malarial work in the U.S.S.R. has been organized on a highly efficient basis. The number of malaria cases has been greatly reduced. The utilization of practical means of control, treatment and prophylaxis has gone a long way in controlling the spread of this disease. Educational work among the masses has also been very effective.

XII

THE CONTROL OF VENEREAL DISEASES

HEALTH in the Soviet Union is regarded as a matter of the greatest importance affecting all the people throughout the country. For this reason public health agencies, hospitals, clinics, etc., have been organized on a highly efficient basis. The village and city Soviets supervise the hospitals maintained on their budget, combat venereal disease, maintain sanitary supervision and have facilities to care for the mentally deranged. The *rayons* or districts have various committees of which that concerned with public health is regarded as among the most important. At a higher level is the People's Commissariat for Public Health which controls the entire health work of the nation.

Among the most notable achievements of the People's Commissariat of Health and the smaller health units of the U.S.S.R. has been the control of venereal diseases in the Soviet Union. Venereal diseases were widespread in Czarist Russia. For example 30 per cent of the Yakut population were infected with syphilis; in Moscow the incidence of venereal disease in 1914 was estimated as 338 per 10,000 of the population. The estimate for the country as a whole in 1913 was 76.8 cases of syphilis per 10,000 population.

Syphilis was spread by various means in addition to the conventional method, such as by feeding babies on pre chewed bread, smoking communal water-pipes, or kissing ikons. Prostitution was still, however, the chief means of spreading venereal infections.

When the Soviets came into power, they began immediately, under Dr. Bronner, a campaign to combat venereal infections. A special Bureau for Venereal Diseases of the People's Commissariat of Public Health was established in 1918 and 1919 saw the Bronner Institute for Skin and Venereal Diseases established in Moscow. This had 440 beds as well as the usual research laboratory and out-patient facilities and had under its administration in the city twelve small institutes and thirty dispensaries. In its first fifteen years 2,800 physicians attended postgraduate courses in venereology varying in length from ten days to four months. A scientific journal was established for the dissemination of information on venereal diseases.

Primarily the organization for combating and controlling venereal disease is based on the dispensary unit. Smaller areas have venereal stations with small staffs and rather simple but adequate equipment. The more outlying rural areas are served by means of mobile units or flying squads whose responsibility it is to diagnose and treat all cases of venereal disease in these districts.

The doctor in charge of a venereal disease dispensary is appointed by the health department; he is specially trained in this work. His duties consist of keeping the scientific work of the dispensary up to date, maintaining strict control and registration of all possible sources of infection, and examining wherever possible all contacts in schools, factories, collective farms, and so forth.

The dispensary staff is organized on a basis of 0.6-0.8 visits per inhabitant served per year, and must consist of at least two medical officers, two *feldshars,* one female visitor, one clerk and two female orderlies. All these dispensaries have facilities for dealing with syphilis and gonorrhea, including separate rooms and separate times for women and children.

Another function of the dispensary is the organization of conferences for workers. Lectures are given on social hygiene. Films, posters and exhibitions are shown in factories, schools, farms, and elsewhere. Courses in sex hygiene are given at regular intervals. Very close touch is maintained with maternity and child welfare clinics. Blood for Wassermann reactions is taken as a routine at prenatal clinics in a further attempt to control venereal diseases.

Much is done to spare the patient's feelings; it is made as impersonal as possible. On the first visit each patient is given a number and no further use of names is necessary. All subsequent visits are made by appointment, the clinic being open from morning until night. All patients in the infectious stage of the disease are treated in the hospital. In spite of the fact that it is a disease caused by misconduct all patients receive full sick benefits. Those who fail to show up for treatment are visited by a nurse who ascertains the reasons for their failure to report for treatment and impresses the seriousness of their illness upon them.

Most nations have realized that compulsion in the matter of treatment is one of the ways to control and combat venereal diseases. In the Soviet Union decrees passed in 1927 and 1929 gave added powers of compulsory and, if need, repeated medical examination of anyone who is suspected of suffering from a venereal disease.

These laws provide that compulsion may be used to secure treatment, and for wilfully and knowingly exposing to infection or infecting another person, there are penalties of from six months to three years imprisonment. However, it is seldom necessary to make use of these compulsory powers, most persons realizing the seriousness of their infection and cooperating to get it under control. There are, however, circumstances when it is necessary to take more stringent steps and isolate the person infected with a venereal disease in order to protect others. These include domestic workers, pupils and wet nurses and others who come in contact with great masses of people.

Patients are further encouraged in helping to combat venereal diseases to bring along for examination the person from whom they contracted the disease as well as members of their own families with whom they came in contact and whom they may have possibly infected. This is most important in controlling the spread of the disease.

Prostitution is still the chief source of the spread of venereal diseases throughout the world. This the Russians know full well. They have always regarded prostitution as being primarily due to economic causes and have dealt with the problem along economic lines. The two most important factors in reducing prostitution in the Soviet Union has been improving the economic status of women and in improving the economic level of the general populace. This latter factor has acted first by making early marriages possible, and second for women to be gainfully employed in most industrial enterprises in the Soviet Union.

When the Soviets took over the country from the Czar, prostitution was widespread throughout the land. First there was established a network of "prophylactoria" over the country. Then began a process of reeducation of the prostitutes so that they could become fit to take part in the industrial life of the country. Also, all infected prostitutes were treated for venereal infections. In Moscow nearly 4,000 women passed through the prophylactoria from 1927 to 1936. Of these nearly 90 per cent were infected with venereal disease, and of this total, nearly 90 per cent have since earned their living in industry, of whom 41 per cent are "shock workers" that is to say, highly skilled.

It has been estimated that there were between 20,000 to 30,000 prostitutes in Moscow in pre-Revolution days and about an equal number in Leningrad. Careful checking in 1928 and 1930 revealed 3,000 prostitutes in Moscow and 800 in Leningrad. This great reduction led to most of the prophylactoria being closed. It has been noted that most of the prostitutes today in these cities are feeble-minded or psychopaths.

The campaigns against venereal diseases in the U.S.S.R. is

HALFTONE PLATES

(Photographs by courtesy of Sovfoto)

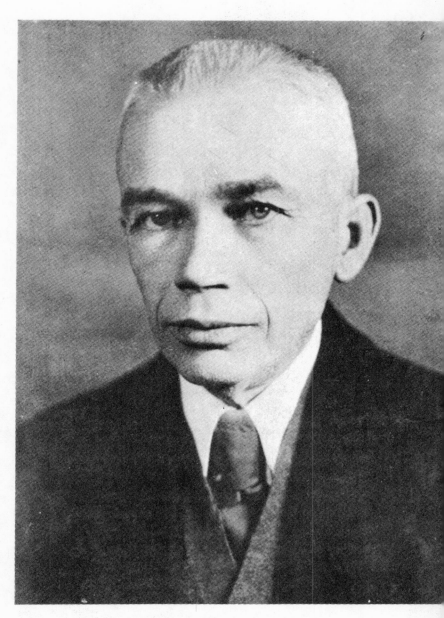

1. The late Dr. A. Bogomolets, President of the
Academy of Sciences of the Ukrainian S.S.R.,
whose experiments in prolonging the life-span
of man stirred interest throughout the world.

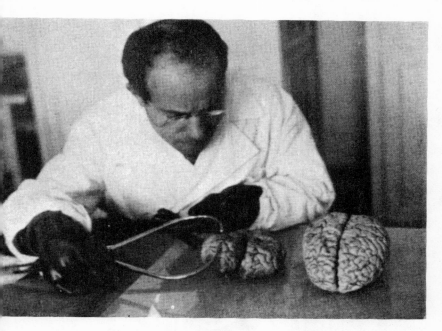

2. Brain studies at Bekhterev Brain Institute, Leningrad.

3. Experiment in which an animal's heart was kept beating after removal from the body.

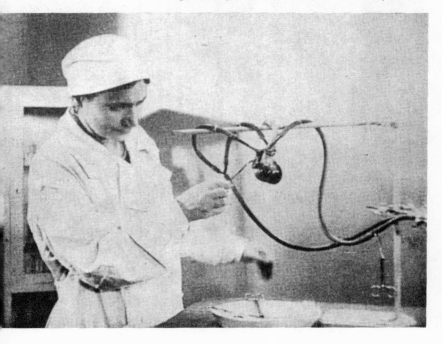

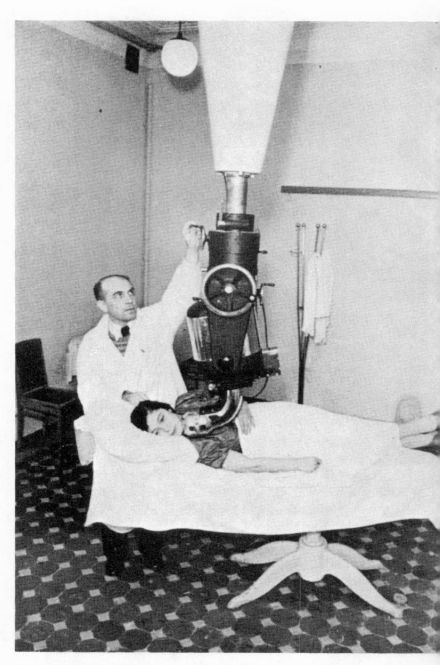

4. Radium-gun in the Central Institute of Oncology,
Moscow, being used to treat a cancer patient.

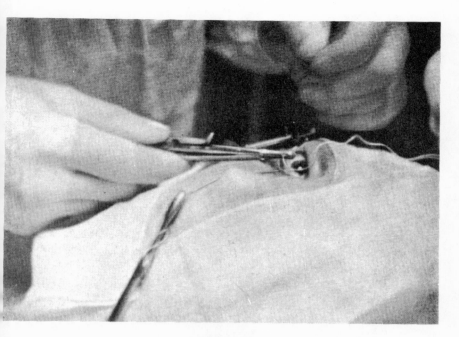

5. Grafting of a cornea, taken from a man recently dead, to the eye of a blind person.

6. A plastic operation on the genitals, being performed by Prof. A. Frumkin (center).

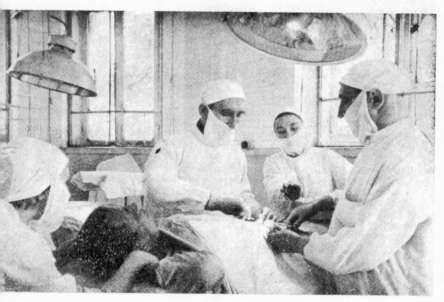

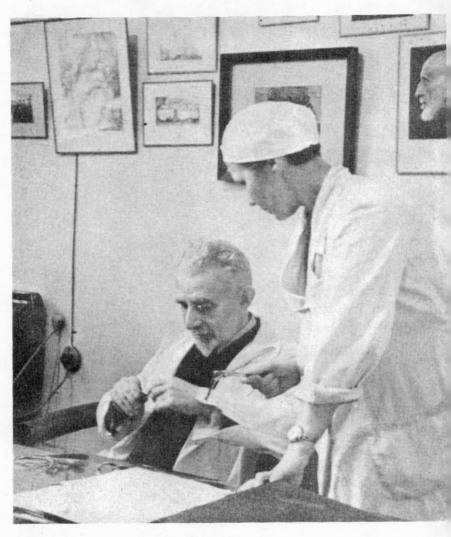

7. Dr. Mikhael Averbach and his assistant, Dr. Eugenia M. Ivanova, testing new instruments designed at the Helmholtz Institute for delicate eye operations.

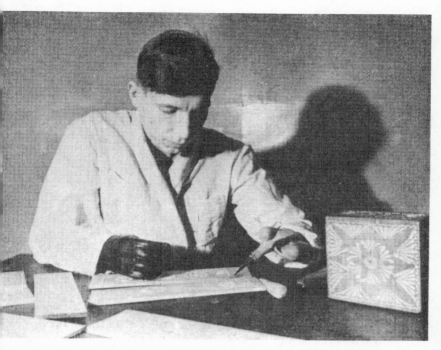

8. This soldier lost both arms, but now has artificial "fingers," made by splitting a forearm. He has become a skilled carver.

9. Valentin Chereponov (right), who had been clinically dead, is shown playing dominoes.

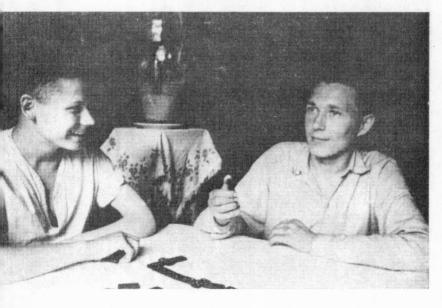

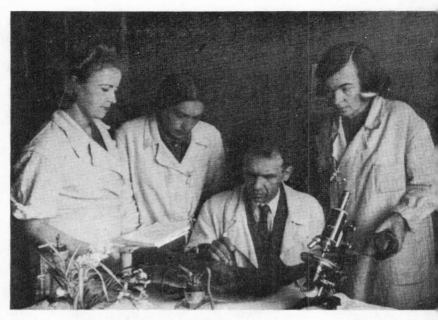

10. **Prof.** Negovsky and his assistants studying a
heart contraction curve.

11. Transplanting nerves from the dead to the
living. Dr. A. Vishnevsky (left) is shown performing a nerve transplantation operation.

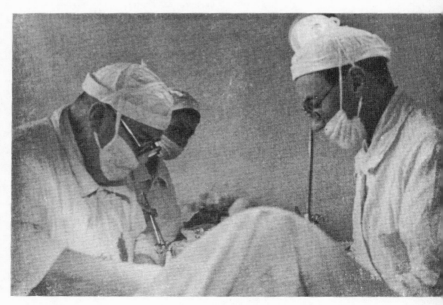

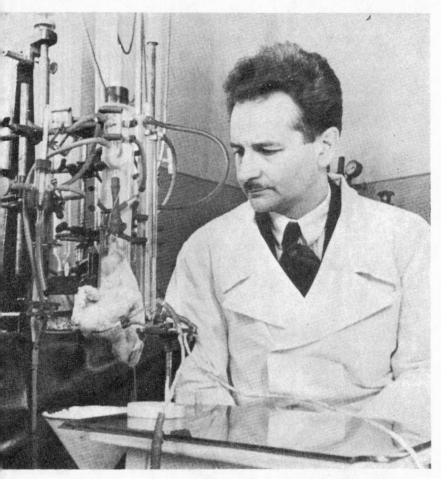

12. Docent S. V. Andreyev, Botkin Hospital, Moscow, is shown experimenting with the heart of a man dead nearly 100 hours.

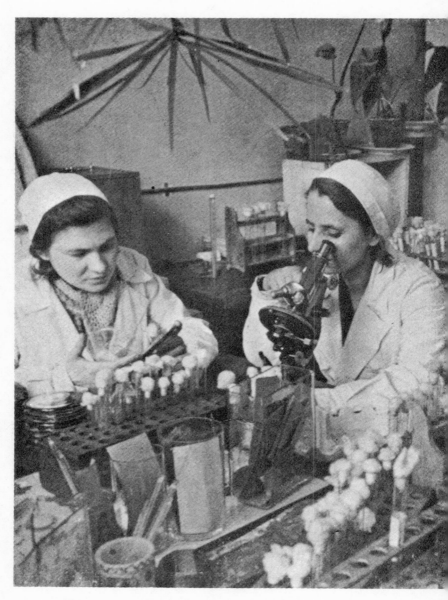

13. In the laboratory of the Botkin Hospital,
Moscow.

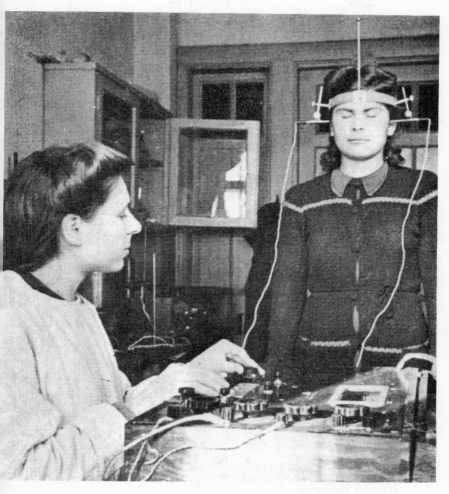

14. Research at the Botkin Hospital, Moscow. A research worker measures the excitability of the patient's vestibular apparatus.

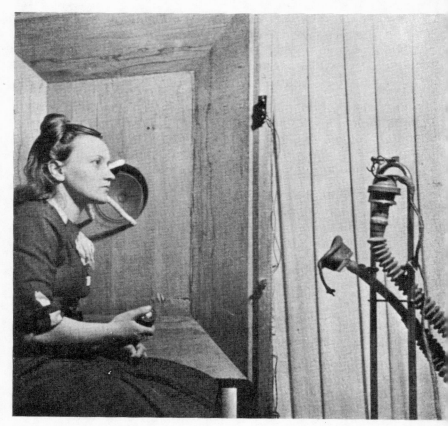

15. The special sound chamber in Prof. Trutnev's laboratory at the Botkin Hospital, Moscow, is being used for hearing tests.

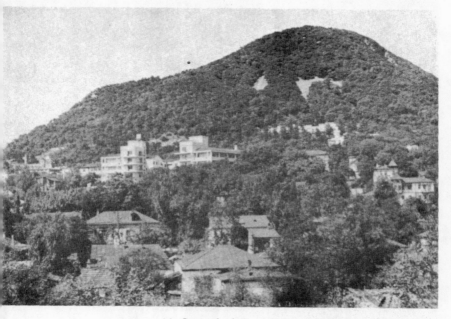

16. General view of the Zheleznovodsk health resort with the Zheleznoya mountain in the background.

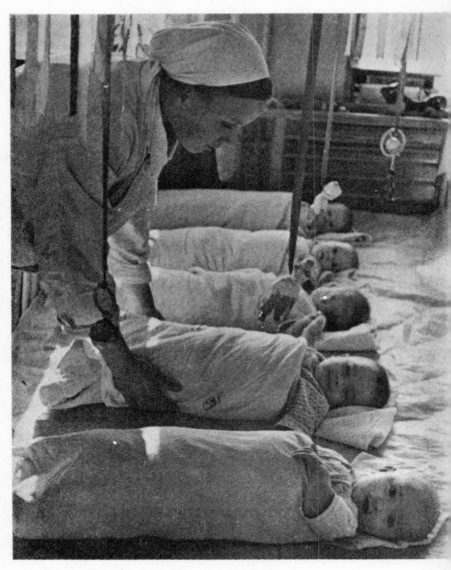

17. These babies spend their days at the nursery
attached to the Kaganovich State Ball-bearing
Factory where their mothers work.

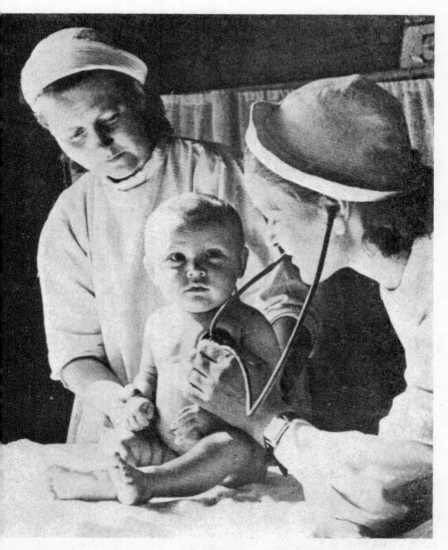

18. Checking up on children's health. Dr. Nadezhda Kudryavtseva examines the youngsters of Ryblovo village regularly.

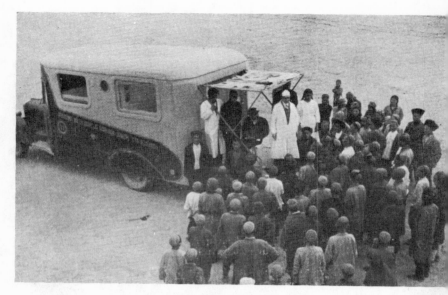

19. A perambulating dispensary for the treatment of trachoma in the Stalin Collective Farm.

20. A nurse from the Women's Consultation Center in Tashkent, capital of the Central Asian Republic of Uzbekistan, visits a factory to lecture on child care.

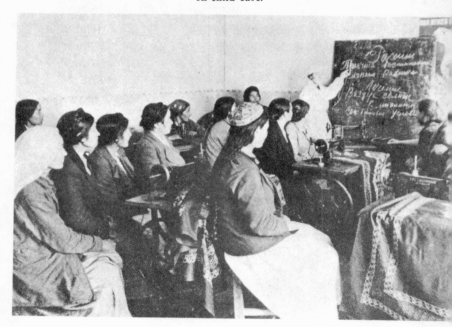

one of the greatest modern achievements in public health. It
is estimated that in the thirty largest cities primary causes of
syphilis decreased by 25.7 per cent in 1939 as compared with
1938. In Moscow primary syphilis is becoming so rare that
medical schools find it difficult to obtain cases for demonstration purposes.

Dyson Carter in *Russia's Secret Weapon*, quotes Quentin
Reynolds' report that Commander Norman, a member of the
Harriman Mission and health officer with the American
Embassy, made this statement: "The Red Army and the Air
Force are virtually free from venereal disease. You can't say
that about any other army in the world. As a doctor that
impresses me."

Dr. J. A. Scott who has made a special study of the venereal
diseases in the U.S.S.R. and who published an article on that
subject in the *British Journal of Venereal Diseases*, March,
1945, has three interesting and significant tables of statistics
which are reproduced here:

TABLE 1
Venereal Disease Dispensaries in Towns and Villages
in the U.S.S.R.

U.S.S.R. and Union Republics	1913	1928	1932	1938	1941
U.S.S.R (Total)	12	800	683	1,351	1,498
R.S.F.S.R.	11	509	412	728	826
Ukrainian S.S.R.	1	206	146	282	295
Azerbaidzhan S.S.R.		10	12	20	21
Byelorussian S.S.R.		14	15	40	38
Georgian S.S.R.		14	16	46	32
Turkmen S.S.R.		6	6	17	21
Armenian S.S.R.		2	2	2	2
Uzbek S.S.R.		14	36	98	121
Tadzhik S.S.R.		..	2	8	9
Kazakh S.S.R.		15	24	75	64
Kirghiz S.S.R.		8	10	26	46
Karelo S.S.R.		..	1	4	5
Moldavia S.S.R.		3	1	5	6

TABLE 2
Number of Patients of Anti-Venereological Dispensaries in Moscow Infected by Prostitutes

Year	Total Patients per 10,000 of the population	Number infected by prostitutes	Percentage of total infected by prostitutes	Percentage compared with 1914
1914	388.7	221	56.9	100.0
1925	190.0	60	31.7	27.1
1927	132.0	35.	26.2	15.0
1934	75.1	9	12.0	4.0

TABLE 3
Reduction in Incidence of Venereal Disease

	Year	Town	Country
Primary Syphilis per 10,000 of the Population	1913	25.7	2.66
	1935	1.8	0.62

First Moscow Dermato-Venereological Dispensary:

Cases per 10,000 of the Population	1923	1932
Syphilis:		
All forms	62.4	34.8
Infective Stage	24.3	4.6
Gonorrhea:		
Acute	61.3	43.1
Chronic	52.7	3.0

XIII

THE ABORTION PROBLEM

ABORTIONS are prevalent throughout the world; in the United States it is still a serious problem which is far from solution. As a matter of fact, the Soviet Union is the only country which made a radical attempt to solve the abortion scourge. At the very beginning of the Soviet regime in 1918, the Soviets legalized abortions, established abortion clinics and performed abortions without charge.

What was the reason for this unusual departure? The reason is very simple: the plan was to protect the health of the great numbers of women who were determined to have abortions. Well known was the fact that secret and illegal abortions were being performed by quacks and midwives under the most unsanitary conditions with the results that there was a very high mortality rate following these illegal operations.

To put a stop to this undercover practice the commissars of public health thought that it would be far wiser to bring this problem out into the open. Abortions were bound to be performed. There was no reason why they should not be performed openly under aseptic conditions, and by scientifically trained medical men who could take precautions and so avoid unnecessary complications.

This plan came into effect during the early days of strife and uncertainty in the new government, a time when disease was rampant, hunger was widespread and suffering was to be seen on every hand. There is now no doubt that this measure saved the lives of thousands and thousands of women.

In 1920 no qualified physician in the Soviet Union could

legally refuse to perform an abortion. However, he could and did discourage the measure. There were certain rules and regulations that had to be observed. Thus, abortion could be refused if pregnancy was more than two and a half months advanced. The patient had to stay in the hospital for not less than three days and was not permitted to return to work until two weeks after the abortion had been performed. Another provision was that an abortion could not be performed earlier than six months following a preceding one. It was noticed that quite a few women had acquired the "abortion habit" and preferred abortion to birth control.

It was not an easy matter to obtain an abortion. Merely requesting it was not an assurance that it would be performed. Following a physical examination, especially a thorough check-up of her reproductive organs by the physician, the patient was visited at home by a social service worker who investigated her economic, social, and living conditions. If the woman could not be persuaded to abandon her plan, a second appointment was made with the clinic physician who again tried to dissuade her. At least 50 per cent of the women were thus dissuaded. If the woman still insisted, however, she was sent to the abortarium where another attempt at dissuasion was made. Here another 25 per cent decided to forego their plans for abortion. As the abortion was performed without the use of an anesthetic only a few were hardy enough to seek a second abortion. There were still those who had acquired the "abortion habit" and still sought abortions, no matter how painful and unpleasant they were.

Here are some rather interesting figures. Out of every 100 pregnant women who came to the Moscow clinics 18 to 20 per cent asked for an abortion. Seventy per cent of those who had no medical reasons for the abortion were dissuaded. In larger cities 40 per cent of abortions were for medical reasons; 44 per cent because of lack of finances or housing; 3 per cent because their work would be seriously impaired; 6 per cent were due to the fact that there were no means of feeding the new baby.

A study of 5,365 cases revealed other causes for seeking an abortion. Poverty was the reason in 31 per cent of the cases; large families in 29 per cent; widows and unmarried women trying to conceal pregnancy in 20 per cent; physical debility, 11 per cent; unhappily married or deserted, 8 per cent.

In 1921 the statistics gathered for the city of Moscow show that six abortions were performed for every 1,000 people. In 1927 it rose to nineteen abortions for every 1,000 people. In 1927 to 1929, 40,000 abortions were performed in Moscow, a ratio of 75 to every 100 births, a truly excessive number. After 1930 the demands for abortions began to diminish in the cities but increased in the rural districts. It was also observed that housewives asked for abortions twice as often as women who were gainfully employed outside the home.

During this period of greatly increased abortions several interesting facts came to light. It was noticed that deaths were very few and less in number than deaths resulting from complications in childbirth. Also infections and injuries to the womb were far less common than they were in illegal abortions. However, other complications were noticed. There was growing evidence of serious organic disorders in women because of repeated abortions. Also noticed were decreased fertility, tendencies to miscarriage, abnormal pregnancies, prolonged labor, endocrine disorders, disturbances in sexual feeling. All these occurred even under the most sanitary conditions. The conclusion that had to be drawn from this experiment in widespread abortion was that interrupting normal pregnancies was not without danger. Abortions were not normal; in time serious disorders would result. The abortion experiment was far from successful.

For this reason, in 1936, the law was modified to permit legalized abortion only when the pregnancy threatened the health of the mother because of the existence of some disease, or because the mother had a disease which could be transmitted to her offspring. Penalties were provided for physicians who broke the law and for husbands who forced their wives into abortion to avoid the responsibility of supporting children. Educational programs were inaugurated to show the danger of abortions to health.

Another measure to counteract the demands for abortions was the expenditure of millions of dollars for maternal and infant welfare. Children in the Soviet Union receive the best of care. From the day of their birth, children are placed under adequate nursery and medical supervision. Millions of children are cared for in kindergartens, day-nurseries, summer-camps and playgrounds.

In 1944 a new law was passed which provides for financial assistance for mothers before the birth of their third and subsequent children. After the birth of the four child a monthly allowance is granted until the child reaches five years of age. The allowance increased with each child after the fourth. A Medal of Motherhood is given to mothers who have raised five or six children. The Order of The Glory of Motherhood is conferred upon the mothers who have raised seven, eight, or nine children, while the first degree award, Mother Heroine, is given to those who have borne and raised ten children.

This is a swing in the opposite direction. Russia realizes that measures to increase the population are of greater security to the nation than those that encourage its decrease. Abortions are no longer free and easy to obtain. Economic conditions have been improved to such a degree that poverty and inability to care for and raise children is no longer a valid reason for obtaining an abortion. Motherhood is now so highly regarded and so amply rewarded that any woman who seeks to avoid it is regarded with suspicion and distrust. Abortions are not so popular as they formerly were.

The law has been changed in regard to abortions in the

U.S.S.R. Under the present law abortion is restricted in about the same way as it is in the United States. Abortion can be performed only for therapeutic reasons; reasons that are concerned only with the health of the mother or the health of the unborn child. Violations of this law are severely dealt with. The Soviet Union is just as vigorously putting down illegal abortions as any other country.

XIV

THE WAR ON CANCER

THE greatest advances in the study on cancer are being made in the United States, Great Britain and the Soviet Union. Some of the most interesting discoveries in regard to cancer have been made in the U.S.S.R. within the past few years.

The fact that there is any cancer research at all in Russia is remarkable when one considers the paucity of cancer work in Czarist Russia. According to I. M. Neuman: "Only a few individual investigators, among whom were N. N. Petrov and A. A. Krontovski, occupied themselves with experimental oncology (cancer research) in Czarist Russia. The single actual attempt to organize an experimental laboratory (in the Moscow Cancer Institute) not only did not lead to the creation of a group of experimental oncologists but the laboratory itself was closed just before the First World War.

"Before the Revolution, there did not exist in our country a single experimental oncological laboratory. At the present time we have scores of laboratories devoting their entire time, or a considerable portion of their time, to problems of experimental oncology. Special oncological institutes, with a number of experimental laboratories, have been established in Leningrad and Moscow. The directors of the experimental work are N. N. Petrov, N. A. Krotkina and N. G. Khlopin and N. V. Okunev in the Leningrad Institute; and A. G. Andres and I. M. Neuman in the Central Oncological Institute of the People's Commissariat of Health of the R.S.F.S.R. in Moscow. Large experimental oncological departments have been organized within the Roentgen Institutes of Leningrad, Kiev, Kharkov and Moscow. Oncological laboratories exist in the All-Union Institute of Experimental Medicine in Leningrad, in Moscow, in the Kiev Institute of Experimental Biology and Pathology, in the Ukrainian Institute of Experimental Medicine in Dniepropetrovsk and in the Sverdlovsk Institute of Physiotherapy, and in the Voronezh Roentgen-Oncological Institute. In Moscow there is the Laboratory of Experimental Oncology. Extensive work in experimental oncology is conducted in the laboratories directed by K. P. Ulesko-Stroganova in Leningrad and G. O. Roskin in Moscow. Oncological subjects occupy considerable time in the work of the chairs of the medical schools."

It is thus seen that cancer research is going on in a great many hospitals, institutes and medical schools scattered throughout the nation. Various aspects of the cancer problem are being studied by scores of medical scientists at the various research laboratories and clinics. The way x-rays and radium act on cancerous growths have received careful attention at the hands of Mishchenko, Petrov and Krontovski. The work of Gurvich has attracted world-wide attention. He has conducted a great many experiments on certain rays given off by tumors, particularly cancerous tumors. These so-called mitogenetic rays have aroused a great deal of interest in the United States. This work is still in the experimental stages and there is much to be learned before any definite statements could be made.

The part that the nervous system plays in cancer has received the attention of Tserniakhovski, Soloviev and others. For instance, Soloviev has concerned himself mainly with the effects of the nervous system on the spread of cancerous tissues and cells in the human body. Tserniakhovski has done some remarkable work in describing the effects of nerve endings when they come in contact with cancerous tumors.

What effect does cancer have on the metabolism or inner

activity of the body? Many problems have been solved in this direction by the brilliant work of Dr. Reprev and Dr. Mishchenko. Another interesting phase of metabolic activity in relation to cancer has been the elucidation of Medvedeva of the alteration in the carbon-nitrogen ratio in the urine. The breathing of respiration tissue activity of cancer tumors as well as of the organs of cancer patients has been investigated by Kavetski.

Interesting and significant work on the chemical properties of cancer cells has been done by Magat who studied the permeability of cancer cells and the effect of acids on cancer tissue. Kaplanski has done considerable work on the protein metabolism of cancer growths.

Dr. Shor has done much to clarify the ways in which cancer-producing substances act. He has described the general effects of the action of coal tar and cancer-producing hydrocarbons; how they initiate and encourage cancer growths. Very interesting experiments have been conducted by Shabad who demonstrated the presence of cancer-producing substances in the liver and other organs of patients with cancer. Extracts made from the livers of non-cancerous patients have been ascertained to have the property of producing cancers in mice.

The old problem of chronic irritation and cancer production has been studied anew by Petrov and Krotkina. Petrov is one of the foremost cancer experts in the U.S.S.R. He has conducted experiments in the production of cancers in rats following the transplantation of embryonic tissue. Dr. Krichevski and Dr. Sinelnikov have succeeded in transplanting cancer from man to rats.

A series of very significant experiments have been carried out by Drs. Khlonin, Timofeevski and Andres on the tissue culture of human and animal cancers. Krontovski has utilized this method of tissue culture in studying the metabolism of cancerous growths. Andres has recorded interesting form changes in the nuclei of cancer cells.

The relation between cancerous growths and the organism in which these growths occur have received careful consideration from many medical investigators. Dr. Roskin has shown that it is possible to transplant cancers from one part of the body to another by merely blockading the reticulo-endothelial system.

Drs. Bogomolets and Kavetski investigated the mechanism of stimulation and blocking in the function of the mesenchymal tissue in the production of cancer. They have shown that anti-human spleen horse serum has the ability to cause the cancer-destroying capacity of the serum of patients with cancer. Drs. Larionov and Iasvoin have demonstrated the importance of aging of the connective tissue in the development of tar cancer.

Careful check is kept upon cancer research going on in other parts of the world. In 1940 they established a special periodical devoted to cancer research, *General and Special Oncology*, which is devoted to a thorough review of the various phases of cancer research all over the world.

The first congress of cancerologists of the Ukrainian Republic was held in 1938 and it was well attended. Many recommendations were made at this meeting which since then have been carried out. Laboratories were established for the testing of various compounds used in industry as possible cancer excitors. Special institutes have also been established for the biological and biochemical methods of treatment and diagnosis of cancer.

How does cancer research compare with that in the United States and Great Britain, the two other leading cancer research countries? It compares favorably with the work in these countries with one notable exception. Very little work has been done in the genetic aspects of the cancer problem.

particularly the work of Maude Slye in the United States. Some attempts are now being made to overcome this deficiency.

However, certain aspects of cancer research have been emphasized in the U.S.S.R. and neglected elsewhere. These have been the effect of cancerous growths on the organism in which they occur and the roles of the nervous system and the reticulo-endothelial system in the cause and growth of cancerous tissues.

Cancer research did not suffer any interruption because of the war. It went on elsewhere when the Germans invaded the Ukraine and other territories. A broad biological view of the entire cancer problem exists and much of great importance has been learned along biological lines about cancer growth and development.

XV

PHYSICAL FITNESS ON A NATIONAL SCALE

PHYSICAL education in the Soviet Union is taken very seriously by all the people; it is organized along national lines. Its ruling body is the All-Union Council of Physical Culture, which is appointed by the Council of People's Commissars and is responsible only to this body. Its membership is composed of experts in physical education and their headquarters are at Moscow.

There are many similar subordinate councils of physical education throughout the U.S.S.R., each separate republic having one of its own. They are, however, subject to the national council at Moscow, whose rules are binding upon all of them.

The chief object of physical education in the Soviet Union is to build a healthy, strong body for a healthy mind. The first requisite is for a constant supply of qualified physical culture teachers. The training of these teachers is the function of the Institutes of Physical Culture. There are several such institutes scattered throughout the country—Leningrad, Moscow, Kharkov, Kiev, Baku and Tiflis. These institutes have certain professional standards and requirements, equal to other professional schools, such as medical, musical, and so on.

The teaching and training at these institutes is most thorough. Sports are studied from all angles. The medical aspects of physical education are thoroughly gone into. Besides pure physical training and conditioning, the scientific evaluation of both the methods and those to whom they are applied receive thorough consideration. For instance, here are some of the purely scientific problems studied in the physical training institutes: The different types of nervous systems which are found in the participants in different sports, judged by their speed and accuracy in striking out letters from the printed page. The relation of personality to body type is evaluated. The effects of training through skiing, running and basketball upon protein metabolism. The mechanical analysis of movements of different types of performers in running and gymnastics. The effect on physical output of caffeine and phosphates. Clinical studies of various types of sports.

An average institute contains the following departments of instruction: Department of Physiology and Psychology, Department of Anatomy, Department of Biomechanics, Department of Chemistry, Department of Hygiene, Department of Pedagogy. The instruction in each is thorough and correlated with all the others.

The entrance requirements are rigid: the candidate must have been graduated with high standing from high school, must have been interested in sports and physical training for many years prior to admission, and must pass a medical and physical examination. The examining committee consists of a surgeon, an internist, a neurologist and an ear, nose and throat specialist. The candidate must be in perfect physical condition. For that reason many more apply than are accepted.

The curriculum of these institutes are as follows: anatomy, physiology, biology, physics, chemistry, physical culture for the masses, pedagogy, psychology, gymnastics, aquatic sports, light athletics, physical therapy, public hygiene, military tactics, art gymnastics which includes folk dancing and pageantry.

There are two types of physical culture graduates. The first of these is the coach, who is a specialist in some sport such as gymnastics, aquatics or field and track. He has received two years of training and may only teach his specialty. The second type of graduate is the regular graduate whose training is much more thorough than that of the coach and who teaches theory as well as practice. His training consists of four years. He is the teacher in the institute and other places where not only physical training is given but education as well.

All physical culture activities have as their object the improvement of the participant. They must be protected from injury and mishap. This task is entrusted to a type of specialist known as sports doctors. These doctors are specialists in sports injuries and their rulings are law in all sports. For example, in boxing only five rounds are permitted. Between rounds the physical conditions of the fighters are thoroughly checked; heart is examined and pulse taken. If an injury is inflicted, it is evaluated at once, and the doctor may stop the match if he feels that the fighter has received an injury which should not be aggravated by further combat.

Physical activity is encouraged among all the people generally by the various sports clubs scattered throughout the U.S.S.R. Many of the parks are provided with outdoor apparatus, such as bars, ropes and ladders, as an invitation for all to use them. Facilities are provided for competitive games such as volleyball, tennis and basketball. Pools are to be found in all parks for swimming and aquatic sports. During the day these facilities are for the children, and at night, after work, the adults take advantage of these provisions.

There are also gymnasia in various cities provided with all types of apparatus for sports and physical training of every variety. They are frequently patronized by most able-bodied men and women. All encouragement is given to use these facilities and many take advantage of them.

That physical exercise should be part of everyone's daily life is the point of view held by most of the people in the Soviet Union. A certain portion of the time must be devoted to some form of physical activity in order to maintain a reasonably healthy condition of the body. This is not done haphazardly. The amount and type of exercise is prescribed by a physical training expert in consultation with a sports doctor.

All exercise is carefully planned and more or less standardized. Thus, exercise is given in factories during recess to increase production. Since the workers are vitally interested in means of increasing production they are heartily in favor of the exercises. The physical education expert, who is called in to devise what forms of exercise are to be taken, takes into consideration the type of work done in the factory, the physical condition of the workers and the facilities available.

There are different types of exercises prescribed for men, women and children and for different periods of life. Thus, the exercises prescribed for pregnant women are commenced in the third month, under a doctor's supervision, and are continued as long as he indicates they may be given. Quite often they are given throughout the whole period of pregnancy. These exercises are carefully described in booklets issued by the Institute for the Protection of Motherhood and Infancy of the Commissariat of Public Health.

Exercises are also prescribed for women following the birth of the child. They are under supervision of the doctor. It has been found that these exercises greatly reduce the need for laxatives, improve the morale of the patient and her general bodily health.

Even infants are given exercises, and these are performed by nurses who have received special training from physical culture experts. These exercises are begun at two and a half months and are continued until the infant reaches nursery school age, at which time the child is given a new set of exercises. A series of observations conducted by the Institute of Experimental Medicine have revealed the fact that these exercises have a very favorable effect on the mental as well as the physical development of the child.

A special type of exercise has been devised for the sick. This is a matter of the utmost importance. Many cases of recovery are hastened by judiciously administered exercises. The ill person's physical condition is much improved after a series of mild exercises and he is ready to return to his normal mode of existence in a much shorter time.

The goal of physical culture in the Soviet Union is expressed by the slogan: "Ready for labor and defense." It is the ideal of the Soviet government that the average citizen should be able to get through with his day's work and be unfatigued. Further, he should have enough energy and physical stamina left for play and amusement.

This has been attained in great measure. The people are enthusiastic about sports; they join in all public festivities. The number of stadia in the Soviet Union is large, and most of the institutes for physical culture have their own stadia. Many of the unions too have their own stadia, and numerous events are given in these stadia on special occasions in which a great many participate.

There are also children's stadia exclusively for children's sports, in which children twelve to seventeen compete in various athletic activities. All these activities are carefully supervised by sports doctors.

In these various ways the physical health of the nation is constantly being improved. There are physical activities for all occasions, and the general public enters wholeheartedly into all of them.

Part Two

THE MIRACLES OF SOVIET MEDICINE

XVI

DR. V. P. FILATOV'S TISSUE TREATMENT

THE transplantation of corneas to blinded eyes is one of the greatest achievements of modern medicine. The name of one man stands out among all others in having furthered and advanced the difficult science of cornea transplantation in the fight on blindness and that name is Vladimir Petrovich Filatov.

At the Ocular Clinic of the Medical Institute of Odessa, Dr. Filatov has solved many of the problems connected with cornea transplantation. He found that the following materials can be used in cornea grafting:

1. The cornea of an eye removed from the body of a person just deceased.

2. The cornea of an eye removed from a person on account of a serious disease or injury to the eye which has not affected the cornea.

3. The cornea removed from a person's other blind eye, when the cornea is transparent and healthy.

Dr. Filatov has found that out of 235,000 blind men in his district approximately half have become blind because of opaque corneas. The cornea grafting operation has attained the highest degree of development in Russia because of the cooperation of the government. A systematic search for the blind of Russia has been started by the All-Russian Society for the Blind and much good has been accomplished in their cases by this cornea grafting operation.

V. P. Filatov, the greatest eye surgeon in the U.S.S.R. was born in the village of Mikhailovska, Penza Province, Central

Russia in 1875. His father was an oculist and early in life Filatov became interested in diseases of the eye and determined at that time to become an oculist. In 1897 he received his medical degree from Moscow University Medical School and for two years following his graduation he served as house surgeon in the eye clinic. Later he became house surgeon in the Moscow Eye Hospital. In 1904 he accepted a similar position in the Odessa Eye Clinic. While here he did much research in eye diseases, diagnosis and treatment, and in 1908 he wrote a paper on cellular poisons in ophthalmology which attracted favorable attention and resulted in his appointment as lecturer in eye diseases at the University of Odessa. He also studied his specialty under masters in such clinical centers as Paris, Berlin, Munich, Vienna and Prague.

In 1911 he became the director of the eye clinic of the Odessa Medical Institute, which position he held until the outbreak of the Second World War and in which institute he developed his revolutionary treatments for serious eye diseases, including that of cornea grafting. He was the first to suggest using the eyes of cadavers for this purpose, a practice which has now been universally adopted.

Dr. Filatov is perhaps the most experienced eye surgeon in cornea grafting in the world today. By 1941 he had performed 1,000 such operations. Eye specialists from all over the world have come to Odessa to be trained by Filatov and his associates in this operation, and now it is being performed in almost every country by Filatov-trained oculists.

His fame in his native land is phenomenal. He is known everywhere as the "professor who restores sight." He is truly one of the great national heroes. He has been the recipient of a great many honors in appreciation of his great scientific accomplishments. In 1936 he was elected a member of the Odessa City Council. The following year he was elected a representative to the District and State Congress of Soviets,

He was also chosen as a member of the Supreme Soviet of the Ukrainian S.S.R.

Other honors have also been heaped upon him. He is Scientist of Merit of the Ukrainian Republic. He has been awarded the Stalin Prize and the Red Banner of Labor. He is a member of the Ukrainian Academy of Science and a member of the Scientific Council of the Ukrainian Commissariat of Health.

Now more than seventy years of age, Dr. Filatov is still active. He is Director of the Institute of Experimental Ophthalmology where he still conducts researches in the pathology, management and treatment of diseases of the eye. He is a revered teacher, encouraging his students in undertaking original research to add to our knowledge of the function of the eye and the medical and surgical treatment of blindness. He is one of the greatest oculists of all time.

In 1933 "tissue therapy" was reported by Dr. V. P. Filatov as a new principle in medicine. This method formerly consisted of using similar tissues transplanted from one person to another. Later, various tissues of animals and plants were introduced into the patient. It was found that under these conditions biogenic substances are formed in the preserved tissues which stimulate healing and regeneration.

Dr. Filatov examined the following tissues for availability as healing agents: cornea, sclera, uvea, optic nerve, retina, cartilage, conjunctiva, mucous membrane of the lip, skin, liver, peritoneum, subcutaneous adipose tissue, muscle, placenta, brain, testis and others. Some of the tissue may be obtained from other human beings following an operation, but most of it is obtained from cadavers. Refrigerated animal tissues also possess curative value.

In addition to grafting or implantation, Dr. Filatov found that it was also possible to inject certain fluids obtained from the human body. Thus, he used the decoagulated blood of a cadaver, the blood from the veins of a placenta, the cerebro-spinal fluid of a cadaver, the fluid from eyes—all preserved under refrigeration. Dr. Filatov also found it possible to use extracts obtained from leaves preserved in darkness. One of the extracts used with success was obtained from the juice of the aloe leaves.

Dr. Filatov has formulated a working hypothesis to explain tissue therapy. Here are his ten statements of the explanation of this theory:

1. Isolated animal and plant tissue undergo a biochemical change when certain unfavorable environmental factors interfere with their life processes. These tissues, deprived of a normal existence, form substances that function as stimulators of biochemical processes. These stimulators, which enable the tissues in question to survive in part under unfavorable circumstances, are called "substances of resistance" or "biogenic tissue stimulators."

2. When tissue fragments rich in these "resistance substances" are introduced into the body, the stimulators affect the tissues of the treated organism by increasing cellular metabolism. They intensify physiologic functions and, in the presence of disease, enhance regenerative capacities and aid in the struggle for recovery.

3. These biogenic tissue stimulators have not yet been defined chemically and so far are manifested only by their effects on living subjects. They are probably related to the biogenic amines.

4. These substances originate also in intact living organisms after exposure to unfavorable but not fatal conditions. This is due to biochemical changes in the structure of the organism which may also affect evolutionary processes.

5. Dr. Filatov considers organic disease as structural changes due to adverse conditions and resulting in the formation of stimulators.

6. Toxemia at first inhibits the formation of resistance

substances necessary for regeneration; later, pathologic processes may accelerate the formation of these biogenic stimulators. The phenomenon of crisis may be interpreted as the sudden appearance of these substances.

7. The introduction into a diseased body of tissue enriched with "substances of resistance" acts by stimulating cellular metabolism and it restores the ability of the cells to discharge biogenic stimulators which are indispensable for the entire organism in its struggle against the disease.

8. The development of biogenic stimulators under the influence of environmental factors is the same for animal tissues as for leaves of plants.

9. It is possible that many biologic, physiologic, and pathologic phenomena may be explained by the hypothesis that "the structural change in living matter consists in the appearance of biogenic stimulators which are produced by injury but not death of living matter."

10. Environmental factors which produce the resistance substances may be varied. It may prove possible to demonstrate the occurrence of factors of resistance by exposing tissues and live organisms to various temperatures, radiant energy, and chemical agents. The effect produced upon animal tissues by refrigeration has been most exhaustively studied. The preservation of plant tissues, such as leaves in darkness, also has been carefully investigated.

Dr. Filatov has used preserved tissues in many different ailments. He has used it in the treatment of various eye diseases, such as certain inflammatory conditions, opacities of the lens, atrophy of the optic nerve, vernal catarrh, glaucoma, trachoma, etc. Improvement has also been noted in the sight of the normal eye.

Tissue therapy has been used in conditions other than eye ailments. Among them have been tuberculous ulcers of the skin and larynx, tuberculosis of the lungs, ulcers of the skin, ulcers of the stomach, contractures of joints, diseases of the peripheral nervous system, bronchial asthma and scores of other ailments.

During the war, tissue therapy was introduced into practice at evacuation hospitals. Among diseases of the eye frequent in war, very good results were obtained in inflammation of the cornea, in ulcers of the eye, and in various affections of the optic nerve. Other wartime affections treated with success by this new method were sluggish ulcers, scar tissues, lumbago, and various disturbances of the nervous system.

The sources of tissues are from human cadavers, various animals and plants. The cadavers are selected from persons who died of non-infectious diseases or from accidents. The material is removed under strict asepsis within ten hours of death, is transferred into a dry, sterile bottle, and kept at a temperature of 2°-4° C. for seven days. At the end of this time any germ life that may have been present has totally disappeared.

Tissues and organs such as skin, testes, etc., are obtained from rabbits, sheep and calves. Biological liquids can be used safely, since they can be sterilized.

Dr. Filatov has been using tissue therapy in diseased conditions for many years with very good results. The highlights of his research in this very interesting field are summarized as follows:

1. Animal and plant tissues which have been removed from the host and subjected to conditions hindering growth undergo a biochemical change. Through this change substances are produced, which appear to stimulate the life processes in the original host.

2. When these biogenic tissue stimulators are introduced into the body, they cause an increase of cellular metabolism and, consequently, an increase in physiological function. In the presence of pathologic processes they strengthen the re-

generative ability of the organism and encourage its resistance to disease.

3. The chemistry of these biogenic stimulators has not yet been determined.

4. Biogenic stimulators may be produced in organisms which have been subjected to unfavorable, but not lethal conditions, and perhaps play a part in the processes of evolution.

5. It may be surmised that the above-mentioned conditions which cause modification of the organism and the release of the stimulators are the diseases which attack the organism.

6. Pathogenic factors at first suppress the release of biogenic stimulators. However, with prolongation and intensification of the disease, these same pathogenic factors may encourage the development of the biogenic stimulators. The phenomenon of crisis in infectious diseases may be explained by this concept.

7. Introduction into the sick organism of tissue rich in biogenic stimulators initiated a process which quickens cellular metabolism, and releases vital biogenic stimulators suppressed by the disease.

8. The conditions and factors favoring the development of biogenic stimulators in tissues vary. Among the best known are preservation of animal tissues at low temperatures and storage of plant tissues in dark places.

9. The development of biogenic stimulators under the influence of strongly unfavorable, but not fatal conditions seems to be a train of all living matter. The biogenic stimulators are the products of live, not dead protoplasm fighting for its life. The tissues which produce them, when in a preserved state, are, doubtlessly viable. These tissues, maintained at a low temperature, reproduce through cell division and can yield cell cultures.

10. Many biologic, physiologic and pathologic phenom-

ena may be explained by the hypothesis of active biogenic stimulators evolved by biochemical reconstruction of living matter under the influence of certain conditions.

There is no doubt that Dr. Filatov's tissue therapy represents a valuable contribution to medicine. The scope of application of this new form of treatment is wide, and thus far it has yielded very encouraging results in a great many diseased conditions.

XVII

THE NEW TREATMENT OF PNEUMONIA

ONE of the most profound students of the role of the nervous system in disease is Dr. Alexei Dmitrievich Speransky. His book, *A Basis for the Theory of Medicine,* available in English, is one of the most original of medical treatises; it has attracted a great deal of attention and is exerting a pronounced influence on certain aspects of medical thinking. According to Speransky, disease is not merely the disorganization of normal processes, but the creation of new conditions unknown to physiology.

Speransky was born December 30, 1887, in what was then known as Vyatka and is now Kirov. At the age of 23 he received his degree in medicine from Kazan State University. His early interest was surgery, and at the end of the First World War he became professor of surgery at Irkutsk State University. After about three years of teaching he decided that his main interest lay in research.

In 1923 Dr. Speransky became associated with Pavlov, the leading physiologist in Russia. The following year he was appointed director of an independent laboratory and soon thereafter assumed an important place in the All-Union Institute of Experimental Medicine.

Speransky's interests lie mainly in the physiology of the nervous system. He was particularly interested in the role that the nervous system played in infectious diseases. It was his belief that many so-called direct effects of infection were in reality a reflection of the disturbed function in the nervous system. He evolved his now famous theory which includes

127

new ideas as to the pathology of measles, malaria, scarlet fever, rheumatism, syphilis and other infectious diseases.

He evolved new methods of treating infections as well as infectious diseases. His treatment consisted of the injection of serum intravenously and then applying his "pumping" method. By "pumping" is meant the repeated withdrawal and reintroduction of cerebrospinal fluid under special circumstances. The results were encouraging. Animals infected with dysentery and diphtheria recovered, while control animals given the same quantity of serum but omitting the "pumping" technique died. These methods were also used in hospitals on human patients in the treatment of scarlet fever, tetanus and cerebrospinal meningitis.

The greatest details were evolved in studying the effects of the disease processes on the nervous system. Speransky devoted all his time and efforts in ascertaining the role of the nervous system in the cause of disease. From numerous data he promulgated the theory that many systemic diseases are the external manifestations of changes in the nervous system. What it amounts to is this. Every infectious disease inflicts some sort of injury on the nervous system. Consequently, we have the direct effect of the germ, virus or germ toxin on the tissues and its indirect effect mediated by the altered nervous system. It is Speransky's contention that every infectious disease produces a specific effect on the nervous system which results in a specific symptom complex. The final result is what Speransky calls "a picture of the disease."

Speransky's life work has been concerned with an explanation of all disease on a neurophysiological basis. In 1929 he published his first book on this theory, *The Nervous System in Pathology*. In 1935 he published his famous work, *A Basis for the Theory of Medicine*, which has since then been translated into many languages and has attracted world-wide attention.

The main theses of this book are:

1. Many disease changes, such as ulcers, gangrene, dental caries and drug rashes, the causes of which have been regarded as independent of nervous influences, have been found to depend entirely on such influences.

2. Other disease processes which do not belong to the first group, such as specific infectious diseases, depend partly on the nervous component for their general state.

His work has been highly regarded by the Soviet Union. During the Second World War he held a very important military position. When hostilities ceased he became the head of the department of pathologic-physiology in V.I.E.M. (The All-Union Institute of Experimental Medicine). He also holds the title of Honorary Scientist of the U.S.S.R.

Within recent years Dr. Speransky has discovered some very interesting facts about lobar pneumonia and has evolved a new and effective method for treating it.

He began by experimental studies on animals, especially rabbits. These experiments were aimed at creating conditions in which the specific changes in separate lobes would be permanent rather than temporary. Since lobar pneumonia generally develops unexpectedly in man, it was necessary to determine the intensity of nervous stimulation that produced deep-seated changes in the lungs.

The preliminary experiments were carried out in Dr. Speransky's laboratories by Drs. S. E. Lebedinska and A. M. Chernukh. Rabbits were given a light, volatile narcotic, followed by an injection of 1-2 c.c. of 10-25 per cent turpentine emulsion. On awakening from the anesthetic the rabbit sat, moved about, but was apathetic and refused food. Later, difficulty in breathing developed and in 18-30 hours the rabbit died. The lung changes disclosed at autopsy resembled those found in lobar pneumonia.

As a result of these experiments, Dr. Speransky concluded that certain nerve disturbances produce constant initial changes in the lung, leading to hemorrhages followed by pneumonia and pleurisy. It is Dr. Speransky's belief that the microbe is not the inciting factor when primary nerve damage leads to profound changes in the respiratory organs.

Dr. Speransky and his associates also studied the spread of infection by bronchial, lymphatic or circulatory routes in relation to the main problem. It was determined that the main damage was done by deficiencies in nerve action rather than by germs spread by these various routes.

The speed of deep-seated lung changes, occurring as a result of damage to related nerves was studied in a second series of experiments by Drs. O. Y. Ostri and G. S. Saltykov. An injection of 1 c.c. of a 10 per cent watery solution of chloramine was introduced into the ear vein of a rabbit. In thirty seconds the animal died, and autopsy invariably revealed waterlogging and bleeding of both lungs. This was expected because of the release of active chlorine which injured the blood vessels and lungs. When a weaker solution was used, the animal survived somewhat longer. With the use of 1 c.c. of a 0.5 per cent solution, the animal did not die or develop special symptoms of lung disease. When 0.2 c.c. of a 0.5 per cent solution was injected into the ear vein of a rabbit no reaction appeared, but when injected into a region below the brain the animal died quickly from massive changes in the lungs. The conclusion that was drawn from these experiments was that the damage to the lungs resulted from damage to the central nervous system transmitted rapidly to the lungs and not from direct action of the chlorine on the lungs.

Dr. Speransky sums up the results of all laboratory work on the causes of lobar pneumonia as follows:

1. Profound changes in the lung occurred as a result of various stimuli acting upon the nervous system.

2. The changes appeared in the periphery of the lung, and their intensity depended upon the nature and concentration

of the stimulus, as well as upon the site and methods of injection.

3. Pronounced lungs changes in animal experiments frequently resulted from mechanical and chemical stimulation in the region of the medulla oblongata and the upper segments of the spinal cord.

4. These changes in the lung may develop within a few minutes. This explains why, for example, clinical croupous pneumonia is not only acute but frequently unexpected, "like a stab in the chest with a dagger."

Dr. Speransky then concluded that treatment must be directed not only at the diseased lung but also at the associated nervous disturbance. Proper healing measures should be aimed at overcoming this nervous manifestation.

The following cases were recalled by Dr. Speransky. Some years ago, in one of the Leningrad neurological institutes, when the surgeon accidentally cut one of the upper thoracic intervertebral ganglia during an operation the patient suddenly died from acute lung disturbances. Within a year a similar case occurred under the same circumstances.

A series of experiments was carried out by Dr. Speransky on dogs, in which the importance of the upper segments of the nervous system was established in the cause of lung ailments. Similar facts were noted in his laboratory some years ago when certain disturbances in the medulla oblongata and the upper segments of the spinal cord were followed by changes in the lungs.

This suggested that treatment of pneumonia in men be directed at the nerve segments involved. Local anesthesia of the regions involved was determined upon. This was found to result in an inhibition of the pathological processes.

The area chosen for intracutaneous infiltration with novocaine is an area between the shoulders on the upper part of the spine. From 60 to 80 c.c. of a 0.5 per cent solution of novocaine is used.

Dr. E. M. Ginsburg was the first to adopt this method and in a period of four years he and his co-workers applied it in a series of 200 cases of lobar pneumonia. During the Finnish War Dr. Ginsburg had another 200 cases in which he used this new method. The results obtained were excellent. Dr. Ginsburg noted that the patient's health invariably improved soon after treatment was given. By the fourth day, cough and expectoration had disappeared completely while pulmonary and other changes had returned to normal.

This treatment, when given early, is usually followed by a drop of temperature by crisis to normal within 18 to 24 hours. No second rise occurs although in some cases a drop by lysis occurs within 48 hours. In a number of cases crisis occurs on the third or fourth day of the disease.

The heart action and general condition improves as the temperature drops, but on occasion this improvement preceded the fall in temperature. This crisis is uneventful and is not accompanied by difficulty in breathing, collapse or slowed heart action.

According to Drs. Speransky and Ginsburg there is every reason to believe that improvement in the lung condition begins as the temperature drops and the general condition improves. X-ray studies show that changes in the lung for the better precede the drop in temperature by several hours. With this new method of injecting novocaine under the skin in the region of the upper spine the curative process begins with changes in the lung substances and as a result of restored nerve function. The convalescent period is therefore shorter.

It has also been found that the speed of recovery lessens the possibility of such untoward complications as lung abscesses, formation of adhesive bands around the lungs and gangrene.

Dr. Ginsburg emphasizes the fact that this new method is not intended to eliminate the use of sulfa drugs. The efficacy of the sulfa drugs has been established, particularly if administered in the early stages of pneumonia. As a matter of fact, it has been found that this new treatment tends to intensify the action of the sulfa drugs. It has been found effective in sulfonamide-resistant cases of pneumonia.

According to Dr. Speransky the rationale of this new treatment is based on the presumed changes in the lung following restoration of normal nerve function. It is evident that this form of treatment is non-specific, since recent experiments by Dr. Ginsburg showed beneficial results in acute and catarrhal pneumonia where repeated injections are necessary. Finally, it has been demonstrated that the treatment aids in the absorption of fluids surrounding lungs affected by tuberculosis.

There are still many things to learn about this new treatment, and Drs. Speranksy, Ginsburg and others are carrying out experimental and clinical studies of its use not only in pneumonia but other diseases of the lungs as well.

XVIII

DR. BOGOMOLETS' ANTI-OLD AGE SERUM

THE most famous of the Russian old-age fighters was Alexander A. Bogomolets, who attracted world-wide attention with his methods of retarding the advances of old age by means of blood transfusions.

Bogomolets was born in prison. In 1881 his mother was incarcerated in the Lubianovka prison because of her revolutionary activities. She was a medical student and before she left for Siberia she gave birth to her son, Alexander Alexandrovich Bogomolets, who never saw his mother. The future doctor was raised by his grandfather, a retired army officer, in the province of Poltava.

In 1906 Bogomolets received his degree in medicine from the University of Odessa Medical School with high honors. He was interested in pathology and upon graduation received an appointment in that department of his alma mater. Within five years his work in pathology attracted wide notice and he was appointed professor of physiologic pathology at the University of Saratov. During the First World War Dr. Bogomolets served as consulting epidemiologist for the southwestern front with great distinction. After the Revolution he went to Moscow to resume his research in disease phenomena, and from 1925 to 1930 he was professor of pathology at the Second Moscow University.

Bogomolets was also interested in the new science of endocrinology which resulted in his publication of the book, *The Crisis of Endocrinology.* He was also very much interested in biological problems as applied to medical research and it was at this time that he was much intrigued with the problems of the causes of old age.

The eager Dr. Bogomolets was universal in his medical interests. He became interested in the functions of the nervous system, and he organized a laboratory at the Moscow Hippodrome for the study of acute neuro-muscular fatigue in horses and the effect of special diets on fatigue.

From his interest in the nervous system he was led to a study of the blood, particularly blood transfusions. This now became his primary interest and in 1924 he helped found the Central Institute of Blood Transfusions which did a great deal of pioneer research in this field. He was also instrumental in the establishments of blood banks in various hospitals throughout the Soviet Union.

While engaged in research at the Central Institute of Blood Transfusions, Bogomolets formulated his theory of colloidoclasia which explains the healing effects of blood transfusions. It was his contention that the colloids in the donor's blood acted upon the tissues of the recipient in such a manner as to expel diseased and defective particles from the cells. This was in the nature of a healing cleansing which accomplished much in bringing about a cure and rejuvenation of the body.

From 1930 Dr. Bogomolets devoted all his energies to the study of the causes of old age. He had moved to Kiev where he became the founder and director of the Kiev Institute of Experimental Biology and Pathology. He published his views on old age in a book, *Constitution and the Mesenchyma*. Here he performed many experiments which upheld his views that the cells of the connective tissues have the properties of intercepting and destroying germs which enter the body. It is these very cells that determine the body's resistance to infection and predisposition to the changes of old age.

With a staff of sixty assistants, Dr. Bogomolets set about to discover means of prolonging human life. This in the main consists of repeated small volume transfusions at regular intervals. His methods are fully described in his book, *The Prolongation of Life*. It is his thesis that the usual span of human life should be from 125 to 150 years, which is five to six times longer than the period of maturation.

The theories and practical applications of these theories in the field of longevity promulgated by Dr. Bogomolets are well known in the Soviet Union and are quickly attracting attention all over the world. In 1938 the Bogomolets Institute in Kiev sent a special expedition of scientists to Abkhazia in the Caucasus Mountains. The object was a field study in human longevity. Twelve persons with ages ranging from 107 to 135 were examined by the doctors of the expedition. All of them were in the best of health, and the youngest of the group, a lad of 107, announced that he was planning to get married again.

It was the opinion of Dr. Bogomolets that these long-lived people are not curiosities, but normal individuals who have managed to live the normal span of human life. The Bogomolets Institute, which is devoted to the study of longevity estimates that nearly 30,000 persons in the U.S.S.R. today have passed the century mark, and that there is no reason why many more thousands should not do so.

Dr. Bogomolets was not only a biological scientist but a social scientist as well. He knows that social conditions have profound biological effects on the human body. He attributes, among other things, the causes of premature old age to social conditions, such as hunger, cold, poverty, poor hygienic conditions, all of which have definite effects on the human organism and render it susceptible to a variety of devitalizing diseases. The use of improper food, the inordinate consumption of alcoholic beverages, the breathing of impure air, all have deleterious effects on health which tend to shorten human life.

It is well known that the major diseases of mankind, such

as syphilis, tuberculosis, typhus, malaria, arthritis, and so on, very definitely shorten human life. Dr. Bogomolets also contends that the minor ailments such as the ordinary cold, infections of the nose, sinuses, tonsils and other very common and ordinary ailments also tend to shorten life.

The first requisite in prolonging human life is to enforce the principles of preventive medicine. The living condition of the people must be improved. There must be a sufficiency of the proper foods. The air must be freed from impurities. There must be moderation in the use of alcohol and tobacco. Ordinary, common sense hygienic measures must be carried out. The prevention of colds and other infections is necessary. Certainly the major ailments must be avoided by the employment of all the preventive measures that modern medicine has to offer.

Dr. Bogomolets arrived at an estimation of the span of human life by examining the length of the period from birth to maturity of various animals and comparing that space of time with the average life span of these animals under favorable conditions. It was discovered that in most cases the animal's life span was five to six times longer than its period of maturation.

Concerning this Dr. Bogomolets said: "Let us assume that this observation is correct. Then, taking into account the fact that the development of the human organism terminates in its basic outlines about the age of 25, it may be considered that the normal life span of man constitutes 125 to 150 years. I think, however, that even this age must not be regarded as the limit."

The main fact that Dr. Bogomolets discovered in his old-age studies is that the physiological system of connective tissues within the human body are of the greatest importance in prolonging human life. It is a well established fact that the cells of the human body derive nourishment from the blood stream through the connective tissue, much in the same manner as plants draw nourishment from the soil through their roots. The total health of the human being, therefore, depends upon the condition of the connective tissue just as the growth and development of the plant depends upon the condition of its roots.

The main principle that Dr. Bogomolets put forth is that since the aging of the human body begins to manifest itself with the aging of the connective tissue, to preserve the strength and health of the connective tissue is of prime importance in the fight against the advances of old age. Working with his son, Dr. Olog Bogomolets, Dr. Bogomolets performed a great many experiments in his institute. Recently he announced: "We in the Institute have found a reliable way of acting upon the connective tissue. We inject a fluid with a rather complicated name, anti-reticular cytotoxic serum."

The effect of this anti-reticular cytotoxic serum is to stimulate the functions of the physiological system of connective tissue. Overdoses must be avoided, as they have been found to have just the opposite effect. When properly administered this serum has been used successfully to hasten the healing of fractures, the alleviation of arthritis of the joints, and as a preventive against the recurrence of tumors after their removal.

There is nothing magical about this serum. It does not banish old age with magical promptness. "It is difficult to change the course of a river," says Dr. Bogomolets. The serum tends to retard the process of exhaustion of the human body, to delay the setting in of senility and to overcome the factors which tend to destroy the connective tissue and thus age the human body prematurely.

Before the war the Soviet government set up in Kiev a Clinic for Combating Premature Aging of the Organism. Here only patients of over fifty were treated. These patients were instructed as to diet and the general principles of health

and hygiene. They were given small injections of the Bogomolets serum. After a course of treatment the health of these
patients improved rapidly. Headaches, arthritis, and other
ailments associated with old age disappeared, and the working
capacity of those treated increased greatly.

At this date there are throughout the Soviet Union, a
great many cases of long-lived people which give every hope
for the success of experiments in longevity. Bogomolets tells
us of the case of a peasant named Shapovsky to whom the
famous French author Henri Barbusse, was introduced when
he visited Russia in 1927. Speaking to this peasant, who lived
in the village of Lati, near Sukhum, Barbusse was amazed to
find that the man was actually 140 years old and still possess-
ing considerable strength and vigor. Shapovsky's third wife
was then 82 years old and his youngest daughter was 26.

Dr. Bogomolets had some definite suggestions for the
average person who has ambitions to prolong his life. His
first principle is *work*. The health of the human body demands that all its functions be brought into activity which
can best be achieved through work. There should be no
abuse of any bodily function through excess of any kind:
food, drink, overwork, etc.

Exercise has a place as a preventative against old age. Ten
to twenty minutes of exercise a day Dr. Bogomolets considers
of value. The metabolism between the tissues and the blood
is speeded up through exercise, and the feeding of the cells is
aided along with the discharge of waste materials.

It is the opinion of Dr. Bogomolets that correct breathing,
which enriches the blood with oxygen, is also of great importance because it burns up harmful toxic substances in the
body. Sleep is another important factor in preventing premature old age. These simple rules go a long way in preserving health and delaying the onset of premature senility.

One of the most remarkable achievements of the Bogomolets Institute has been a series of experiments with what they

call the "hormone of rest." This hormone when used properly in the elimination of fatigue accomplishes wonders in prolonging life. The fighting of fatigue is one of the objects of modern medical science today. This hormone, derived from the adrenal glands, is of definite value in preventing fatigue and all its devastating effects.

In an article by Dr. Bogomolets, *On the Therapeutic Action of the Anti-reticular Cytotoxic Serum*, he summarizes the actions and effects of his serum in the following words:

"I would compare the action of our serum, though I wish to stress that this is merely a comparison, with the action of a match causing a conflagration. I think that autocatalysis is the basis of the stimulating action of anti-reticular cytotoxic serum. Small doses of the serum, penetrating the histocytic elements, stimulate the production of substances which actively affect their functions. It may be supposed that these substances are secreted by the blood and lymph and that they subsequently stimulate specifically the cellular elements of the connective tissue system.

"We may think, or perhaps it is better to say, we hope, that the anti-reticular cytotoxic serum proposed by us, which already has proved a powerful means for mobilizing the plastic and protective energy of the physiologic system of the connective tissue, may also serve to prolong the physiologic activity of its trophic functions. In that case the serum will provide a means of fighting the precocious senile fading of the body, of fighting for its normal longevity."

XIX

SOME ACHIEVEMENTS OF SOVIET MEDICAL RESEARCH

MEDICAL research in the Soviet Union has been and is being carried out along a score of different fronts. Special hospitals, clinics and laboratories have been built and equipped for specific types of research and staffed with specially trained medical personnel to direct and carry out this research.

The state encourages the search for new medical facts and techniques. The men who achieve results and discover new methods of combating disease are honored as national heroes. The names and achievements of many of these Soviet doctors are known widely throughout the world. In this chapter will be described some of these significant accomplishments in medicine and surgery.

In the U.S.S.R. the potentialities of skin grafting are taken so seriously that a special supply service has been inaugurated. The required human materials are taken from those who have been condemned to death or are supplied by those generous persons who have willed their bodies for this purpose.

Reparative surgery has now reached magnificent heights in the Soviet Union. The work of Dr. Filatov in grafting new corneas from corpses on the blind corneas of the living has attracted world-wide attention. Similarly, the use of skin from the dead for healing the wounds of the living has now become widespread.

A collective farm woman arrived from the country with a face monstrously eaten away by ulcers and devoid of all

141

emotion and expression. The face was like a hideous mask. Cutting away one of the ulcers, the surgeon replaced it with a piece of skin from a healthy area. Within a few days the patient's largest ulcer had closed up. The resistance of the tissue to the action of the bacteria had strengthened. A struggle had begun in every cell; the ulcers closed up, the inflamed condition was improving and life-giving forces vitalized the skin.

Another worker burned his arm with molten lead. The arm was paralyzed and covered with scars. New skin was grafted on this arm, the scars began to fade away, the tissues became elastic, and the arm regained its flexibility and strength.

Skin grafting is now one of the most highly developed branches of reparative surgery. It is used in filling in voids and helping extensive wounds to heal. Usefulness is restored to limbs contracted by extensive scar tissues, and ugliness caused by disease and accident is corrected.

Severe curvature of the spine is not only a disfiguring disease; it is a disabling one as well. The bone surgeons had been attracted to this problem in bone dynamics for a great many years, and various methods of overcoming spine curvature have been devised.

The first method of overcoming spinal distortion was by means of various jackets and supports. At most, they gave but temporary relief; the curvature, if at all severe, was little affected.

Later, various operations were devised in which added strength was given to the weakened spine by inserting strips of bone in artificially made grooves. Some degree of lessening of the curvature was attained; most gratifying was the relief obtained from pain.

Within the past few years a very remarkable operation for the treatment of hump back has been devised. Professor Kouslick, head of the Orthopedic Clinic of the Central Institute of Traumatology at Leningrad, has discovered a new method for operating on hump backs, by which the chest cavity is not mutilated although the ribs which cause the hump are straightened and realigned.

Twenty-five patients with maladjustment of their spinal columns were treated by Professor Kouslick. In no case was there a fatal result. At the end of the fourth or fifth day the patients could sit up; from the tenth to the fourteenth day they could walk, and at the end of one month or six weeks they could return to work.

The speed of recovery is due to the fact that the chest cavity is left intact. Another advantage of Professor Kouslick's method is the straightening of the trunk. Even very considerable distortions become practically imperceptible under the clothes, and in less serious cases the hump disappears completely.

Into a Moscow hospital a few months ago walked a thirty-year-old woman who complained to the examining physicians that her throat was causing her intense pain.

When her throat was examined it was found that there was a band of contraction about her larynx. Questioning her, the doctors learned that she had suffered from diphtheria and was about to choke to death from the false membrane that this disease produced in the throat when her doctor made an external opening to enable her to breathe. After the operation had been performed, suppuration had set in and the cartilage around the larynx had begun to disintegrate.

The patient was sent to the Prosthetic Institute in Moscow where Dr. Rauer, the famous throat specialist with the assistance of Dr. Joseph Bokstein, decided to give her a new throat.

This was accomplished by transplanting the cartilage taken from the body of a person who had just died, the operation being carried out in four stages at monthly intervals.

Eventually the larynx was completely restored and, at a recent meeting of the Moscow Surgical Society, Dr. Rauer revealed that the woman now equipped with borrowed cartilage had a new throat which had proved very satisfactory in every respect.

Blood transfusions and other uses of blood have received widespread attention in the U.S.S.R. Many interesting studies have come from Soviet hospitals, laboratories and clinics concerning the miracles that may be performed with blood. Dr. Bogomolets has done remarkable work with blood transfusion in delaying the onset of old age.

Dr. Bogomolets' theory as to how blood transfusions help in rejuvenating the system is most interesting. Since the aging of the organism is accompanied by accumulation within the cells of biologically inert protoplasmic molecules, their removal from the cellular elements by means of blood transfusion must have, to a certain degree, a rejuvenating effect on the organism. It is possible, therefore, according to Dr. Bogomolets, for small, frequent transfusions to delay premature aging of the body.

The resorptive effect of transfused blood suggests the possibility of favorable action of blood transfusion in functional disturbances of the blood vessels, according to Dr. Bogomolets. It is therefore possible that repeated blood transfusions may prove an effective measure against the development of arteriosclerosis.

Two other Soviet scientists who have done much with blood in the treatment of various conditions are Drs. A. A. Bagdasarov and M. C. Dultsin. They have found that blood transfusion in large doses produces a healing effect in hemophilia (bleeder's disease). Blood transfusions are of value in treating infectious diseases because they lead not only to a higher degree of non-specific immunity, but also to non-specific desensitization and detoxication. Blood transfusions are also of value in vitamin deficiencies. Small doses of blood create a favorable "soil" for more rapid and effective use of vitamins and minerals.

Blood products, particularly thrombin, have been found by Soviet neuro-surgeons to be of great value in operative work upon the nerves and brain. Dr. N. I. Propper-Grashchenkov stated: "In the nerve clinic of the All-Union Institute of Experimental Medicine at Moscow, which serves the seriously wounded in skull, brain, spinal column and spinal cord, since the end of April, 1942, thrombin prepared by V. A. Kudryashov has been used as a hemostatic agent in operations on the brain and spinal cord. In all cases there was a definite effect on the duration of bleeding from the small vessels of the brain and the tissue of the scalp and spinal column."

Soviet medical men have done much with blood. They have developed blood thrombin, a chemical powder very effective in stopping bleeding from the most serious wounds. Extracted from blood, it can be sprinkled on the brain to control diffuse bleeding. Because it is a natural substance, there is no danger in leaving it in the body after an operation since it is absorbed.

Fibrinogen is another product derived from blood. A little like nylon, it can be made in the form of sheets, powder, sponges and strings. It has the power of clotting blood and absorbing it, and later being absorbed itself. Fibrinogen sponges are left inside the body without harm. They stop bleeding from serious wounds in an amazingly short space of time.

Red blood cells, an important by-product of plasma production, are made into a paste which speeds healing of old, infected burns, varicose and other ulcers, and extensive granulating wounds.

Some interesting discoveries about human radiant energy have been made by Soviet scientists. Dr. Gurwitsch, of Leningrad, states that he discovered that blood as well as the brain, nerves and other parts of the body actually emanate specific types of rays, generally known to scientists as mitogenic rays,

life rays, or M-rays, which lie in the ultra-violet portion of the
spectrum. They are given off from plants, yeast and similar
living organic structures. All organs of the body, he says,
have their own specific biological spectrums.

Dr. Gurwitsch has found that as soon as cancer begins to
develop, the normal spectrum of the blood, as mentioned
above, undergoes a change. This change is definitely a warning signal that should be taken seriously.

Another Soviet scientist, Dr. D. N. Borodin, maintains
that so far twenty-five biologic spectrums have been mapped
out by Dr. Gurwitsch and himself. These include two specific
spectrums for cancer.

"It is interesting," states Dr. Borodin, "that spectra of
cancer tissues are not identical during the different stages of
the disease." Cancer is different at different stages of its
development so far as ascertaining it by these waves are concerned. This is a most interesting discovery and later may
prove of great value in conquering this disease.

Painless childbirth through hypnotism has been another
achievement of Soviet medical men. Professor V. Zdravomuslow of the Moscow University School of Medicine has been
the pioneer in developing this new method of making childbirth easier and less painful.

The story of Professor Zdravomuslow's first attempts at
obstetrical anesthesia by hypnosis goes back to 1925 and it
has now developed to a high stage of perfection. This is how
hypnosis is used today in childbirth. A few weeks before
birth is expected, the mother is prepared by a course of
hypnotic training. In some cases, however, the specialist
inducing hypnosis starts the treatment during the actual
labor when the pains first begin.

Complete success is obtained only when freedom from pain
is produced during the whole of the period from the com-
mencement of pain until delivery. Success is considered to
be only partial when the pains, though considerably reduced,

are not completely eliminated; failure, when hypnosis has had but little effect. Positive results have been obtained in 88 per cent of all cases, of which one half respond fully during the entire duration of labor.

The length of preparatory training varies according to the suggestibility of the patient and the depth of the subsequent hypnotic sleep. Pregnant women who respond favorably to suggestion attend for hypnotic treatment at intervals of from one to two weeks, sometimes even dispensing with the training period altogether. Others have preparatory treatment every two or three days, and sometimes even daily in certain cases.

During this hypnotic training period, two aims are kept in mind: (1) to dispel the conviction that pains are unavoidable and put the patient in a peaceful frame of mind; (2) to endeavor by oral suggestion to diminish sensitivity to painful sensations which may in spite of everything occur by reason of the abnormal distention of the tissues.

The first objective is easily obtained in almost every case. After a few treatments those who are dreading what lies before them are calmed and no longer afraid.

The use of psychotherapeutic analgesia is spreading among hospitals and maternity clinics in the Soviet Union. The only difficulty with hypnotism is the great amount of time that the specialist must be prepared to spend, and the enormous expenditure of energy that he must make. But it is almost always found that the results fully compensate for the initial effort.

From Moscow has come news that Professor Sinitsin, of the Gorky Medical Institute, succeeded in transplanting the hearts of frogs. Professor Sinitsin had to develop a method for rapidly sewing up blood vessels, and his first series of experiments enabled him to place a second heart inside the animal's own heart. Later, he cut out the hearts of certain frogs and placed transplanted hearts into their blood-vessel

systems. Transplanted hearts functioned normally, some of
the animals living for 100 days. They did not show any
difference in behavior from normal frogs, and they mated and
spawned in the spring.

Continuing his experiments Dr. Sinitsin then transplanted
hearts through frogs' mouths, the animals' own hearts being
removed at the same time, and the "new" heart immediately
included in the blood-vessel system. There was a minimum
loss of blood by this method, and at the time of Dr. Sinitsin's
reports, some of the frogs had lived for 130 days. Cardio-
graphs of the transplanted hearts coincide with those of the
unoperated ones.

Valentin Cherepanov was dead. The surgeon made entry
in the case history: "Death following shock and acute hemorrhage on March 3, 1944, at 14:41."

Valentin Cherepanov would have remained dead had not
Soviet medical science formulated methods of combating pre-
mature death from wounds. Formed ten months ago by the
Red Army Medical Board and the People's Commissariat of
Health, the brigade was headed by Vladimir Negovski, di-
rector of the Laboratory of Experimental Physiology of the
All-Union Institute of Experimental Medicine.

Three and a half minutes after death had been recorded,
the group went to work on the body of Valentin Cherepanov.
One minute later Cherepanov's heart began to beat and, after
three minutes, respiration appeared. Within half an hour
he had recovered consciousness. Then he fell into a doze. His
name was called and he opened his eyes and answered questions. He asked for a drink. His breathing was even and his
pulse regular.

Today Cherepanov feels perfectly well, but he is under
observation at the All-Union Institute of Experimental Medicine. Dr. Negovski and his co-workers Drs. Smienskaya,
Litvinov and Kozlov have already tested their methods on
fifty-one officers and men with severe injuries to the internal

organs or limbs. In all these cases the usual means of saving
life had failed. In twelve wounded men the vital functions
were restored and the patients later treated for their wounds.
In the other cases the return to life was brief, lasting only a
few hours or days.

Briefly, Dr. Negovski's method of revival is as follows:
(1) oxygen is supplied to the lungs directly by a pulmotor,
and (2) blood is introduced not only into the brachial vein,
but also into the artery, in the direction of the heart. This
method restores nourishment to the heart muscle. Dr.
Negovski's method is simple and readily available.

Dr. S. V. Kravkov has been doing original research on the
stimulation of vision for the past several years. He found that
the problem of sharpening visual functions may be reduced
to the application of external stimuli and the use of medicinal
agents. Moderate light stimulation of the eye was tested as a
means of increasing the light sensitivity of vision. The following facts were disclosed. If in the course of dark adaptation the visual field is illuminated with a light of moderate
brightness for one to five minutes, at further stages of
adaptation, the eye will exhibit a higher degree of sensitivity
than it could reach without such stimulation. An appropriate
dosage of additional light stimulation produces a significant
and durable positive effect with rather rare exceptions.

Various drugs, Dr. Kravkov has found, are also capable of
beneficial influence on vision. Strychnine pills have been
used with great success in improving visual sensitivity. Experiments were conducted on twelve subjects. All showed
that the injection of strychnine produces a considerable and
protracted intensification (lasting two to three days) of the
discriminative power of the eye.

XX

THE RECALL TO LIFE

MAN hates death. For thousands of years he has fought against it. The desire for life is so strong that many methods have been evolved to prolong life just a bit longer in spite of the greatest obstacles. So old is this struggle that the first trials to overcome death are mentioned in fairy tales, myths and popular legends. Even before the medical triumphs of the ancient Greeks, there are recorded attempts to bring back life by transfusing blood into the lifeless. Similar experiments were carried out by the priest-doctors of the Greeks and Romans.

Some thirty years ago Ilya Mechnikov, the great Russian physiologist, wrote: "It may be presaged that the study of death in plants, animals and human beings will reveal data of supreme interest to science and mankind." He differentiated between two types of death. One was the death which comes as a result of senile changes in the organism and the other is the premature death which comes as a result of accident and disease.

According to prevailing concepts, life is a special form of protein organization developed in the course of evolution. In accordance with this concept death assumes a new relationship to life. The study of natural death, the problem of aging, and the possibility of prolonging the natural span of life is one of the problems of modern physiology, as we have seen in the work of Dr. Bogomolets.

Some years ago Drs. Robinson and Shellong observed the beating of the heart thirty-five minutes after the patient was clinically dead. In a number of cases Dr. Fogelson was able to obtain a heart tracing one hour after death. All this means that clinical death is not actual death and that something may be done, in some cases, to restore the human body to life. Dr. Andreyev stated: "A careful analysis of the collapse of the organism reveals that the functions of the medulla (part of the nervous system) and the heart may be reduced to the point of complete disappearance but may still be capable of entire restoration."

All these interesting and very important facts led physicians to the belief that the early stages of clinical death are not final in themselves and that they may be reversed. Again to quote Dr. Andreyev: "All the data pertaining to the continued existence of tissues and organs raise the question of the possibility of reversing the process of dying."

According to Dr. V. A. Negovski, the Soviet doctor who has done the most remarkable work in recalling the dead to life, in the stage of dying, one must differentiate between two connected phases. The first stage is that of agony which is not as the name implies, pain and agony, but the active struggle of the dying body to fend off death. The second stage is that of clinical death, which is a passive condition. Here the heart and lungs have ceased to function but not to such a complete state that biological or final death has ensued. The final stage is true biological death in which all living functions in the body have come to a complete and final stop.

These stages are not always clearly defined and separated. There are times when it is difficult to distinguish between agony and clinical death since the onset of the latter is quite variable and depends upon many different factors. For example, in man, for all practical purposes, clinical death comes about when the blood in the brain ceases to circulate. It is quite apparent that revival is much easier during the agonal stage than during clinical death. Death is very rarely a complete and sudden cessation of life. It is a process involving many intermediate stages from life to death. The closer to life the stage in which the attempt at revival is made the greater are the chances of success.

The first doctor to revive the human heart was Dr. Kulyabko who on August 3, 1902, resuscitated the heart of a three-months-old baby who had just died of pneumonia. Dr. Kuntz in 1936 experimented with the revival of 127 hearts from adult men dead from various diseases and was successful in reviving only 65. He made the observation that the hearts of those who had died from tuberculosis were reactivated easily whereas hearts of patients who died from heart disease were difficult to revive. Since then many successful attempts at reviving the heart after death have been made by various doctors throughout the world.

After many experiments the conclusion was arrived at that arterial infusion of blood with adrenalin and glucose together with powerful artificial respiration is the most effective method of revival. Dr. Shkolvski in 1940 reported three cases in which this method was used with complete success. During the Finnish War Dr. Aizman recalled two soldiers to life by using this method. In 1944 the case of Valentin Cherepanov attracted world-wide attention.

Dr. V. A. Negovski has carried out a long series of experiments in revival of organisms in the state of agonal and clinical death. These experiments were executed in great detail and much of great value was learned which later found practical application. From these carefully conducted experiments the following facts were learned:

1. Revival must begin within a period of five to six minutes after clinical death.

2. In clinical death not exceeding five to six minutes, spontaneous breathing begins usually two to three minutes after revival, when the heart is already functioning. Weak breaths gradually give way to deeper ones, and finally the respiration resembles gasping.

3. The eye reflexes appear seventeen minutes after revival. The earlier the onset of spontaneous breathing the earlier the eye reflexes return.

4. The use of early artificial respiration is very important. "A delay in beginning artificial respiration," say Drs. Towell and Remlinger, "may result in death or survival with profound brain disturbance." Artificial respiration not only increases the oxygenation of the blood but also awakens nerve impulses to the respiratory center. Even when blood is injected directly into the veins, revival of spontaneous breathing will not occur, unless artificial respiration is initiated, and the sooner this is done the greater are the chances for revival.

5. The level of blood pressure at which the first stage of revival proceeds is an important consideration. If the blood pressure is low, spontaneous respiration is delayed. This delay sharply reduces the chances for survival. It is thus important to raise the blood pressure as soon as possible.

6. The moment for intravenous blood injection must be gauged properly. Prolonged intra-arterial infusion, not only delays spontaneous heart action but sometimes leads to its arrest. When artificial respiration is started, intra-arterial injection is stopped. This is a very important point that must be kept in mind.

In successful revival, various factors have to be taken into consideration. Says Dr. Negovski: "Much stress is laid on blood transfusion and artificial respiration in reviving a dying organism, but hithertofore insufficient attention has been devoted to simultaneous, combined action on both bloodstream and breathing. These basic vital functions are so closely connected with one another that isolated attempts to restore either one or the other are insufficient."

Dr. Negovski brings about revival as follows: Air is introduced into the lungs by direct pressure through a tube in the mouth and not by the usual method of expansion and compression of the chest. The expanded lungs excite nerve impulses to the brain, helping the brain cells to revive and assume function. The injection of blood is into an artery and against the blood stream, and not, as ordinarily, into a vein. This sends the blood directly into the vessels feeding the heart and thus restores heart action. After the heart has begun to beat the transfused blood is introduced into the veins.

Time is an important consideration in recalling the clinically dead to life. Revival must be started within five to six minutes after death, before the disintegration of the brain cells have begun. This gives the physician his opportunity for success because once the brain has disintegrated death becomes complete and irrevocable.

After a great deal of research Dr. Negovski is confident that the fighting time against death may be extended. "We want to establish exactly which tissues die sooner and which hold out longer, and to determine why they behave in their own peculiar ways. We want to find out everything there is to be known about the mechanics of death so as to be able to fight it. Our work at the front and the young lives we have saved to date are the best spur to further research."

XXI

SOVIET MAGIC WITH BLOOD

THE use of blood in various conditions of the human body characterized by one defect or another has yielded some very remarkable results at the hands of Soviet doctors. They have used blood from sources and for purposes previously not employed and the outcome has been most gratifying.

In 1927 Dr. V. N. Shamov became very much interested in the question of correcting bodily defects by using tissues taken from the dead. He performed a great many experiments to determine the suitability of using different types of tissues and organs from the dead. He particularly became interested in ascertaining whether blood from cadavers could be used in living human beings. He tested the vitality of the blood from human cadavers to replenish the blood volume of dogs nearly dead of exsanguination. The dogs made good recoveries, provided that the blood was taken from ten to twelve hours after death.

Dr. S. S. Yudin applied Dr. Shamov's experiments in human beings, the first case being an engineer who tried to commit suicide by cutting his arteries and nearly bleeding to death. His life was saved by Dr. Yudin who used the blood from a man who had been dead three days. The engineer recovered promptly. Dr. Yudin had six more cases of blood transfused from a cadaver to a living human being before he wrote up his results in a paper and reported them for the first time on September 7, 1930. In November, 1932, he reported favorable results in his first one hundred cases of using blood from the dead to give added years to the dying. Since then this practice has been widely used in the Soviet Union.

The use of placental blood (blood derived from the afterbirth) has been fully developed by Soviet surgeons. The first series of experiments along this line was by Dr. M. S. Malinovski who reported his results in 1934. Two years later, Drs. Bruskin and Farberova of the Central Oncologic Institute of Moscow reported that 114 transfusions of placental blood preserved six to ten days had been used with very good results. Their clinical work had been preceded by many experiments on animals and laboratory investigations of the properties of this type of blood. They were able to recover 50 to 120 c.c. of blood from each placenta.

Within a year Dr. Stavskaya had greatly improved this method. She was able to collect from 80 to 300 c.c. of blood from each placenta and stored the blood for fifteen days. In 1935 Dr. Kantorovich began to use placental blood for massive transfusions and other doctors soon adopted this idea.

Dr. A. A. Bogomolets has used blood transfusions for the treatment of various infectious diseases. Blood transfusions in such infections as rheumatic fever produce desensitization as well as an increase in natural resistance. The effect of blood transfusion in certain forms of pneumonia not only desensitizes the patient and increases his resistance, but also promotes absorption of the exudates produced by the disease, making breathing easier. It is Dr. Bogomolets' belief that small, frequent (200 c.c.) transfusions may delay premature aging.

Dr. Rodigina has had some interesting experiences with the use of blood transfusions in treating eye cataracts. The work in this field thus far is rather limited, but the future holds much of promise.

Drs. A. A. Bagdasarov and M. C. Dultsin have also had wide experience in using blood transfusions in the treatment of infectious diseases. In severe scarlet fever, transfusions of 100-150 c.c. of blood in the first days of illness lead to rapid improvement in 70 per cent and not infrequently aborts the disease.

Excellent results have been obtained by blood transfusions in dysentery. During the early days of the illness, 75-100 c.c. of blood is given and is increased in the later stages to 250 c.c. when anemia develops.

Soviet physicians are using blood transfusions in the treatment of malaria when there is a resistance of the body toward treatment with anti-malarial agents and in the presence of anemia and colitis. In acute rheumatic fever intramuscular injections of blood are given in order to increase the effect of large doses of sodium salicylate. Dr. Goriaev is using transfused blood to which has been added sodium salicylate with very good results.

In cases where fresh blood is not available, Dr. V. I. Kasanski has been using frozen plasma as a blood substitute. The frozen plasma is thawed out in twenty minutes and injected in the usual fashion. Dr. Kasanski has found that frozen plasma after thawing does not show any toxic effects when used in human beings, even in large doses. The healing effects of transfused thawed blood plasma is the same as that with fresh plasma. Thawed plasma may be used for the same diseases and in the same doses as fresh blood. Frozen blood plasma, like fresh plasma, is the best blood substitute.

Dr. Kasanski has found new uses of red blood cells which were formerly discarded when making plasma. He uses the red blood cells suspended in a special solution devised by himself. This liquid is particularly of value in acute blood loss, in septic diseases and anemias due to profuse bleeding.

Thrombin was discovered in the blood about fifty years ago, and until recently little use was found for it. The development of a technological process for large-scale isolation of thrombin was started by Dr. V. A. Kudryashov and his associates several years ago and was perfected by 1943.

Thrombin is now widely used in medicine and surgery.

Dr. N. N. Burdenko has used thrombin in stopping hemorrhage in brain tissues, meningeal vessels and adjacent tissues. Dr. N. I. Propper-Grashchenkov and his associates have used thrombin as a hemostatic agent in operations on the brain and spinal cord. In all cases he found there has been a definite effect on the duration of bleeding from the small vessels of the brain and the tissues of the scalp and spinal cord.

Dr. F. M. Lampert has become an enthusiastic user of thrombin and in a recent article he wrote. "Already in 1942 I was using thrombin in routine operations, especially on tumors, and have always found it to be a valuable agent for stopping hemorrhage. At present I use thrombin not only during operations, covering the bleeding surfaces of tissues with gauze moistened with thrombin, but I usually finish the operations, after suturing the skin, by injecting thrombin into the subcutaneous space and into the tissue cavity by introducing the needle of the syringe into one of the spaces between the sutures. I consider thrombin to be an invaluable preparation which considerably helps to stop hemorrhage and assures complete hemostasis. Thrombin does not produce any untoward action."

Dr. V. K. Trutner, on the basis of numerous operations, reported: "In every case the application of thrombin gave good results. Thrombin is part of our regular practice. It is not contraindicated in the presence of other medical agents or preparations, being entirely compatible with them; it facilitates operation by improving the visualization of anatomic relations and pathologic changes."

The use of incompatible blood is usually avoided under ordinary circumstances. However, Soviet physicians have found that incompatible blood can be used with certain healing effects. Repeated injections of very small doses, five to eight c.c., preferably at intervals of three to four days produce a rather severe reaction, not severe enough to threaten life but sufficiently pronounced to increase the functional activity of the reticulo-endothelial system which is concerned with fighting disease. This type of transfusion has been used with pronounced success in the treatment of chronic or recurrent ulcers of the stomach and duodenum and sub-acute septic states.

A great deal of fundamental work has been done in the U.S.S.R. dealing with the use and action of blood transfusion in various diseased conditions. The use of incompatible work, particularly, has attracted a great deal of attention. Soviet doctors have been performing and are performing veritable magic with blood.

XXII

ACCOMPLISHMENTS OF SOVIET HEART DOCTORS

THE study of heart disease has reached an advanced stage in the Soviet Union; the contributions of Soviet medical men to the science of cardiology have been of the greatest importance. Some of these discoveries have been taken advantage of throughout the world. Others are still in the experimental stage and the further development of these are awaited with the greatest interest.

The nervous mechanism of heart action has been the chief interest of Dr. Lavrentiev for many years. He has found that there are many hundreds of tiny nerves distributed throughout the heart that have not as yet been explored and catalogued. These tiny bits of nerve tissue play a very important part in heart disease. Dr. Lavrentiev has found that in coronary artery disease there is an overabundance of nervous tissue in the heart due to nervous system overactivity. In diphtheria Dr. E. N. Kvodriavtseva found that the nervous tissue of the heart undergoes degeneration.

The effects of various drugs on the heart has attracted the attention of many Soviet heart specialists. Digitalis has received particular attention. Dr. Lang noted a decrease in the excessive blood volume following the use of this drug. In diseases like angina pectoris Dr. Abdulaev found that digitalis is not to be used as it has a tendency to bring on an attack.

Other drugs have also been studied. Calcium has been used to slow down excessive heart action; magnesium to speed up slow heart action. Benzedrine has a tendency to stimulate the heart.

The chemistry of the heart muscle has received a great deal of study. It has been found that acetylcholine and doses of strophanthin increased the glycogen content of the heart; caffeine and large doses of digitalis decreased it, while the lactic acid content of the heart rose. Small doses of strophanthin also promote the utilization of lactic acid by the heart.

The study of arteriosclerosis has been a favorite one among Soviet heart specialists. Especially noted in this line is the work of Dr. Anitschkov who found that cholesterol plays a very important role in the production of certain types of hardening of the arteries. In the specific field of hardening of the coronary artery, Drs. Obrastzov and Strazhesko have found that typical heart tracings can be obtained when there is a hardening of these specific arteries of the heart.

The pain of coronary occlusion has been shown experimentally to be due to distention of the coronary artery with stimulation of the vegetative nervous system and not to spasm. This work was the work of Dr. Shprit.

High blood pressure has been a very fertile field of study. There are many theories advanced to explain high blood pressure. Dr. Kogan-Yasny is of the opinion that the endocrine glands cause the blood pressure to rise. Drs. Konchalovsky and Tareyev believe that constitutional factors are responsible. Dr. Speransky who is primarily interested in the nervous system naturally believes that there is a nervous element in back of the high blood pressure picture. Dr. N. A. Tolubeeva and her co-workers, from their clinical study of individuals with and without high blood pressure, believe that hereditary and traumatic emotional factors are of great importance in the cause of high blood pressure.

It has been ascertained that the eating of too much fatty food has a tendency to keep the blood pressure up. Dr.

Strazhesko is of the opinion that overactivity of the sympathetic nervous system and imbalance of the related endocrine glands produces an elevation of the blood pressure.

Clinical studies have been conducted in attempting to lower high blood pressure. Among the newer drugs tried has been salsolin, a derivative from a native Turkmenian plant, sour-cabbage. The results are uncertain; Dr. Kiskachi believes that this drug lowers the blood pressure, but Dr. Abramova has failed to get any results. Drs. Vasiliev and Latmanizova have had patients inhale negatively charged atmospheric ions and have reported reductions in the blood pressure. Drs. Meizlich and Porkhonik have found that the injections of distilled water lowered blood pressure for long periods of time.

Other types of organic disease besides the three main types, rheumatic, hypertensive and arteriosclerotic have been studied thoroughly by Russian cardiologists. Drs. Veil and Kogan have paid particular attention to emphysema heart. Drs. Ariev and Tigi have studied the heart in various infections such as typhoid fever and brucellosis which cause a slight enlargement of the heart.

The war has drawn attention to heart wounds and their treatment. Dr. Kamenchik has found that even when surgery was accomplished early, within four hours after the injury, the mortality was 50 per cent, in the acute cases. Late surgery, however, in those who survived the acute period, resulted in 47.7 per cent recoveries. Dr. Gamaleya favors conservative treatment, as do most Soviet heart specialists. There have been cases of foreign bodies in the heart without symptoms for as long as twenty-seven years.

Soviet heart men are more interested in the spa treatment of heart ailments than are American cardiologists. There are a great many resorts and mineral spas spread around the Black and Caspian Seas. These are used for the treatment of cardiac patients as well as for their convalescence. Drs. Sokolov and Valedinsky from the Central Institute of Climatotherapy in Moscow list the following as suitable for spa treatment:

1. Rheumatic fever and coronary thrombosis eight months after all acute manifestations are gone.

2. Rheumatic and syphilitic (specifically treated and without angina) valvular disease.

3. Arteriosclerosis and thromboangitis obliterans without gangrene or other acute manifestations.

4. Late subacute thrombophlebitis.

5. Moderate high blood pressure.

Spas are not used for cases of nervous heart disease which improve more readily from travel, sea baths and local physical measures; marked high blood pressure; moderate or severe angina; acute coronary occlusion; cardiac asthma; heart failure—all these require hospital care.

Even finer selection is made by certain Soviet heart specialists. Thus:

1. For pure cardiovascular cases carbon dioxide baths are used.

2. For luetic and arteriosclerotic heart ailments, hydrogen sulphide waters are found especially good.

3. For post-thrombophlebitis cases—mud and thermal baths have been found to be beneficial.

Hydrotherapy in the management of heart disease has been thoroughly studied in the Soviet Union. In Odessa, especially, at the All-Ukrainian Balneo Physiotherapy Institute, the healing virtues of sea-baths and of artificial carbon dioxide baths have been studied, both clinically and experimentally. Dr. Sribner noted increases in the stroke volume, skin reddening and circulating blood volume, and decreases in blood vessel tone and circulation following carbon dioxide baths.

There is no doubt that some very important researches are

going on in Russia today on the causes and treatment of various forms of heart disease. New drugs are being evaluated, new types of treatment are being tried and, in time, some very important advances should be made known throughout the world.

XXIII

TRANSPLANTED HEARTS

THE All-Union Institute of Experimental Medicine in
Moscow is the greatest medical research institute in the
Soviet Union. The great majority of significant discoveries in
medicine in the U.S.S.R. have come from that institute. One
of the most startling of these medical discoveries is the successful transplantation of hearts into warm-blooded animals,
such as rabbits, cats and dogs, which has been accomplished
by Dr. Nikolai Sinitsin.

The first series of the heart transplanting experiments consisted of transplanting the heart into the animal's neck which,
of course, was most accessible and easiest to perform. The
heart was then put in circuit with the animal blood circulatory system. The animals suffered no ill effects as the result
of this transplantation.

The next step consisted of carrying out long-term experiments in which these animals, now having two hearts instead
of one, were kept alive as long as possible, the normal heart in
its regular place and position functioning in unison with the
new, transplanted heart in the animal's neck. These experiments were successful in the majority of the cases, Dr. Sinitsin
reported.

The next step beyond this was to transplant the second
heart into a position in the body approximating the location
of the animal's own heart, namely in the abdomen instead of
in the neck. This was accomplished in many cases with very
good results.

What is the object of the heart transplanting experiments?

There are two, according to Dr. Sinitsin. The first is to get a better and clearer understanding of the physiology and mechanism of the action and behavior of the heart under various conditions. The second is the treatment of various forms of heart disease.

"The transplanted hearts retained their own individual rhythm which as a rule is slower than that of the host's heart," reported Dr. Sinitsin in a report written for a medical journal. "This is significant in that the new, transplanted heart was able to act in a normal, physiologically sound manner and aided in the circulation of the blood. The fact that the new heart acted slower than the old one is also of importance in that it means that it may be possible for the new heart to take over the activity of the old, diseased one in time."

These experiments being carried out in warm-blooded animals, such as rabbits, dogs and cats, and the fact that there was but a very small loss of blood is of the greatest importance. It means that the operation is not a dangerous one and that it may be tolerated without shock or hemorrhage. Another important fact that Dr. Sinitsin observed is that there was no effect on the original heart of the animal. This means that the animal's own heart can continue to function until such time when the new heart is ready to take over the total task of carrying on the circulatory activity of the body.

It was further observed that the operated animals suffered no general ill effects of any kind. There was no shortness of breath, spasms, or excessive excitation of any kind following the operation. Also, they reacted in a perfectly normal manner to all external stimuli, such as light, sound and pain.

This latest work of heart transplantation of Dr. Sinitsin is a logical follow-up of earlier experiments in which he succeeded in transplanting hearts in cold-blooded animals. In these earlier experiments, the transplantation consisted in replacing one frog's heart with that of another frog. These experiments had been carried out for a number of years and careful records were kept.

It is a matter of record that some of these frogs lived more than six months with the new transplanted heart. They did not show any differences in behavior from normal, one-hearted frogs. In the spring both males and females which had been operated upon went through a normal mating period which ended with spawning.

"Microscopic examination of the blood vessels that had been sewed together showed that they had knitted completely and that the structure of the heart muscles was normal," Dr. Sinitsin reported. This demonstrated that the new heart and associated blood vessel system was able, in a comparatively short time, to become a physiological part of the animal's body and take part in the bodily functions without acting as a disturbing element. This fact is of the greatest importance in that it means that the transplanting of a new heart into the body does not mean a radical departure from usual bodily activity and function. It means that it is possible to transplant hearts and for these hearts to assume normal activity.

Also says Dr. Sinitsin: "When there are two hearts beating in the breast of one frog, they have entirely different relations to the animal's body. The host's own heart has both neural and humoral connections with his body through the blood while for the first thirty-five to forty days the transplanted heart has only humoral and chemical connections." This is also a fact of great importance. It means that the new heart does not at once undertake the function of the old heart and thus cause a profound disturbance in the physiology of the body. The new heart has an action all its own, apart from the animal's own heart. It functions in a perfectly normal manner for a transplanted heart, while new connections are being established slowly and in a perfectly normal and orderly fashion. There is no clashing of activities of one with the other.

Continues Dr. Sinitsin: "The nerves of the host then begin to grow onto the transplanted heart. It is also possible to study the action of a number of heart medicines on the organisms with two hearts." In time the new heart establishes nerve connections with the body and is beginning to take on true heart activity, just as the animal's own heart. It is beginning to gain strength and activity more in the nature of the heart's work of pumping the blood in an orderly, normal, rhythmical fashion. The effects of various heart medicines on an animal with two hearts is a new source of information of how various heart remedies act and is of the greatest importance in the treatment of heart diseases.

"There is undoubted interest in the question of the length of time taken by a transplanted heart to take root in the host's organism, when the host's nerves grow onto it and what happens to nerve ganglions inside the heart," writes Dr. Sinitsin. This is a very important question which will be answered in time by careful studies in dissections of the two-hearted animals. Time is still required to reveal the answer to this important question, and when the answer is obtained it will add a very important bit of knowledge to the physiology of the heart and heart action.

Dr. Sinitsin continues: "The success of these experiments on cold-blooded animals led me to repeat the experiments on rabbits, cats and dogs. As a preliminary measure we carefully developed methods of joining blood vessels of warm-blooded animals. The method we developed is exceedingly simple and rapid, taking twenty to thirty seconds to perform." Speed and simplicity is of the greatest importance in all blood vessel surgery. The object of preventing blood loss and shock is then attained. This is even more important in heart transplantation work. The speed of the operation is mainly responsible for the survival of the operated animal. The attainment of a speed of twenty to thirty seconds is phenomenal.

"For the first series of these experiments we developed

methods of transplanting the heart onto the necks of these animals. In this series of experiments the second heart had only its right half joined into the host's blood circulatory system. The last half of the heart was not 'in circuit.' This system we called the 'semi-clinical' method.

"Observations showed that the heart worked well and would live for a long time. The heart retained its own rhythm and had no adverse effect on the blood pressure of the host to his ability to perform work." This is an indication of the completely successful working of the new heart in its new surroundings. The retained rhythm of the heart means that it suffered no ill effects and that it was able to carry on its function without altering the blood pressure and related body functions.

"For the second series of experiments after a long search for the correct method we transplanted hearts onto necks of hosts with both halves of arterial and venous in circuit with the blood circulatory system. This gave us a complete 'clinical transplantation.' "

These later experiments gave more complete data on the function of the new heart. There is every indication to point to some new and startling future discoveries using heart transplantation not only to study heart activity but also to ascertain new and revolutionary methods of treating the No. 1 killer, heart disease.

XXIV

SOVIET GRAMACIDIN

WITHIN the past few years several new anti-biotic germ fighters have come into existence, the most famous of these being penicillin. However, other fungi have been found to possess germ-killing properties, among them streptomycin and gramacidin. Among the most powerful of the gramacidin group is Soviet gramacidin or gramacidin S.

It was during the summer of 1942 that G. F. Gause, chief of the department of microbiology of the Institute of Tropical Medicine in Moscow, and M. G. Brazhnikova, research fellow in the department, undertook a systematic investigation of various strains of antagonistic sporulating bacilli from Russian soils. Among several hundreds of isolated strains they studied, only one culture isolated from a garden soil showed high germ killing activity. This strain, after a great deal of investigation, was called after the discoverers the Gause-Brazhnikova strain and served as the source of a new and very powerful germ killer which was named gramacidin S.

The first of the members of this new group of germ killers, tyrothricin, was isolated in the United States. It was found that gramacidin S is somewhat more effective in killing staphylococci, whereas tyrothricin is more active in killing streptococci and pneumonia germs. Both together therefore become a very effective germ killer against all three types of germs.

Another advantage of gramacidin S is that it is not accompanied by any increase in toxicity when compared with other germ killers in its group. It was further ascertained that concentrated solutions of gramacidin S do not interfere with the activity of the white blood cells in human wounds when applied locally or in cavities. Dr. L. Levinson of the Histological Laboratory of the University of Moscow recorded the favorable action of gramacidin S upon healing tissues in wounds and noted particularly the increase in cells rich in nucleic acid.

Another advantage of gramacidin S is its great stability. The dry crystalline form does not lose its germ killing properties even after it has been heated to 160° C. Even when hydrochloric acid is added to a watery solution of gramacidin S it still retains its activity.

Gramacidin S has been found useful in treating wounds infected with the most dangerous germs. Lacerated wounds of muscles in guinea pigs infected with gas bacilli and treated with a water solution of gramacidin S healed successfully. The mortality of animals treated with gramacidin S was 5 per cent whereas in untreated animals it was 53 per cent.

It has now been definitely established that gramacidin S represents a new substance of biologic origin which possesses great germ killing action against many bacteria. It is more universal in its anti-bacterial action than any similar agent and it is entirely harmless when applied locally which is not true of similar germ killers. Gramacidin was admitted by the Medical Research Council of the U.S.S.R. for wide medical use in July, 1943. It has proved its great value in a great many hundreds of cases.

Gramacidin S is distributed in ampules containing 4 per cent alcoholic solution of the dry substance. It is stable, in this form, for at least two years. A feature possessed by gramacidin S and not by others in this group is that it alleviates pain in many instances.

Gramacidin S has been found valuable in the treatment of infected wounds and ulcers of various kinds. In infections of soft tissues, severe burns and abscesses this germ killer has acted with remarkable results. Many cases of prolonged suppuration of six to eight months duration responded well to gramacidin and were completely healed in from twenty to thirty days. Dead tissue disappeared and was replaced by healthy, live tissue in all these cases.

In preparing surfaces for skin grafting gramacidin is proving of the utmost value. The wound surface is abundantly irrigated by a watery solution of gramacidin S before and after transplantation of skin grafts, and in all instances the results were favorable.

In osteomyelitis gramacidin S is now used in helping accelerate the healing process. Recovery is possible in many cases without further suppuration.

In empyema and peritonitis the application of a watery solution of gramacidin S renders the pus sterile, kills all germ life within the area and accelerates healing. Recovery thereafter is rapid and most satisfactory.

In various skin diseases gramacidin is used in either a watery solution or in the form of ointments. Dr. P. G. Sergiev treated 117 patients with contagious impetigo with an alcoholic solution of gramacidin and the period of recovery averaged four days. In twenty-three patients with more deeply seated injuries of the skin, the period of recovery was six days. Seventy per cent of chronic suppurations of the skin that had lasted from three months to three years were completely cured within sixteen to thirty-one days.

Drs. A. A. Manevich and G. Z. Pitskhelauri also used gramacidin S in a large number of cases. They found that slow-healing infected wounds and ulcers responded favorably in three to four days. Pus, together with foul odor, disappeared and were replaced by brand new healthy tissue.

A special characteristic of gramacidin is its ability to act in the presence of pus and other secretions, unlike that of the sulfa drugs. Applied locally, gramacidin is not poisonous and does not irritate the skin around the wound.

Ulcers of long standing which do not yield to other agents heal rapidly and cleanly without any ill after-effects when gramacidin is used. Indolent granulation tissue, resistant to usual methods of treatment, become activated after gramacidin.

Cases of extensive eczema which are usually resistant to treatment heal quickly when gramacidin is applied locally, followed by irradiation with quartz lamp.

Gramacidin S has been used in several thousand cases throughout the Soviet Union and its efficacy has been thoroughly established. Chemically it has been determined that gramacidin S represents a new crystalline polypeptide which differs from both the American gramacidin and tyrocidine hydrochloride.

The following facts about gramacidin S are summarized briefly:

1. Gramacidin is a biological antiseptic which is highly bactericidal. It is capable of killing many varieties of germs on mere contact.

2. It is not injurious in concentrations of 0.4 to 0.8 mg. per c.c. of aqueous solution. It does not prevent bacterial action by the white cells or, to use the technical expression, leukocytosis. It is effective against streptococci as well as against staphylococci, the two most common varieties of germs causing infections on the surface of the body as well as within the body.

3. It does not lose its power or potency in the presence of pus, as so many other germ killers do. It does not irritate wound tissue or tissue around the wound and thus does not interfere with the natural processes of healing. It acts favorably on regeneration of the wound tissues as well as epithelialization, the growth of new cells.

4. The longer the cultures are under the influence of gramacidin, the better is its action. No toxic results are mani-

fested no matter how long the gramacidin may act upon the cultures.

5. The more serious the wound infection, the higher must be the concentration of the solution.

6. It has been found that the best results are obtained with irrigations for a period of three to four days or daily wet dressings.

7. In later stages of wound healing, gramacidin emulsion or ointment may be used, changing the dressing every other day.

8. The powdered gramacidin and alcohol solutions are stable for a long time; the water solution must be prepared on the day of use.

9. Gramacidin produces deleterious effects on the red blood cells and for this reason cannot be used intravenously or even locally when bleeding tissues are present.

10. Gramacidin has found wide use in the treatment of purulent wounds, chronic ulcers, osteomyelitis and some forms of skin diseases.

11. Gramacidin quickly prepares infected wounds and ulcers for plastic surgery.

XXV

NEW METHODS OF TREATING SHOCK

SHOCK is one of the greatest killers in accident and disease. It is also the worst feared of all complications following a serious operation. During the late war shock killed as many soldiers as bullets. It is one of the greatest problems in medicine today. Many physicians have been studying shock throughout the world and many interesting facts regarding it have come to light. In the U.S.S.R. shock has been claiming the special attention of a group of specialists, among them Dr. E. A. Asratyan who has evolved a new method of treating shock.

Just what is shock? Shock is a profound disturbance of the entire body resulting from a disturbance and weakening of the basic nerve centers. The blood vessels of the entire body are primarily affected. The coronary circulation, the blood supply to the heart, is profoundly affected. There is also a loss in tone of the arterioles and capillaries. The blood oozes out of these small blood vessels and stagnates. Profound biochemical changes take place in the entire body; all important functions are upset and in many cases death results.

Dr. Asratyan undertook a series of experiments to investigate the various phenomena associated with shock. These experiments were directed along the following lines:

1. The functional restoration of the disturbed nerve centers.

2. The restoration of the tone and function to the disturbed arterioles and capillaries.

175

3. The neutralization of the various toxic substances that are formed during shock.

To accomplish the first of these objectives, that of restoring the function of the nerve centers, Dr. Asratyan decided to follow the observations of Dr. Pavlov to emphasize increased physiological rest by inducing sleep. The experiments were directed first at slowing down the central nervous system and prolonging sleep in shock patients by the use of sedative and hypnotic drugs. This was not a new departure.

The various sedative and hypnotic drugs in common use were tried and found unsatisfactory. A new drug or combination of drugs had to be evolved. At length, after many trials, Dr. Asratyan compounded a solution made up of fourteen grams of sodium chloride, 2.5 grams of calcium chloride, 1 gram of sodium bicarbonate, 1.2 grams of sodium bromide, and 20-24 grams of glucose. These were dissolved in 40-45 c.c. of distilled alcohol and 1,000 c.c. of distilled water. Primarily, this solution was designed to remain longer in the blood stream, to restore tissue fluids and red blood cells to the blood stream, to increase thirst, to hasten water and salt metabolism, and to stimulate the kidneys.

Each of the compounds used in this physiological solution has a definite purpose. For instance, calcium chloride raises the tone of the blood vessels and diminishes water-logging of the tissues. It helps to strengthen the capillary walls and to improve heart action. The sodium bicarbonate helps to overcome the acidosis which is present during shock. The sodium bromide induces relaxation. The sugar and alcohol have a soothing and anesthetic action and help to induce restful sleep. They also have a stimulating effect on the inner bodily processes as well as a nourishing action.

After more experimental work, Dr. Asratyan selected a drug known as hedonal as the hypnotic drug best suited for the treatment of shock. This drug is the least harmful of all the hypnotics and the best acting and small doses may be used to obtain the desired results.

Armed with these therapeutic measures, Dr. Asratyan conducted a series of laboratory experiments on animals in which he produced shock by various traumatic methods. Shock was manifested by the following signs: Blood pressure fell to about 20-30 per cent of the initial level and bodily temperature dropped markedly. Breathing, heart action and nerve action were all markedly depressed to a dangerously low level. Half of the animals were treated with the new solution and half were left untreated. Those that were untreated died.

Those that were treated survived. Administration of the new solution brought about the following changes. Soon after its introduction, there was a gradual rise in blood and pulse pressure. Circulation and breathing improved; the blood became bright red and its coagulability increased. About ten minutes after the infusion, the animals gradually relaxed and then fell asleep. Pulse and breathing became normal. Upon awakening one to two hours after treatment, they drank eagerly, stood, walked and ran like normal animals.

Following these experiments, Dr. Asratyan began to use this method in the treatment of shock in human beings. The first treatments were given in the emergency hospitals of Tashkent. Later, it was tried in various mobile hospitals at the front lines. Data was collected in a series of 110 patients treated by this new method.

Only two of the 110 cases treated with the new solution did not respond favorably, but the others all reacted well. In general, three to five minutes after the infusion was begun, the pulse was able to be felt, and soon became steady and rhythmic. Blood and pulse pressure rose quickly, reaching normal levels toward the end of the infusion, an increase usually of 50 to 60 millimeters. Pallor gradually disappeared, the pupils contracted, and the breathing returned to normal rate, rhythm and amplitude. Sensitivity and motor activity were restored.

Shortly after the treatment, the patients began to become aware of their surroundings, to stir and to complain of pain. They talked willingly about their wounds, but felt better and were calm. Within twenty minutes they gradually became sleepy and fell into normal sleep lasting two to four hours, during which the blood pressure fell a few millimeters and the pulse became somewhat irregular. Both the pulse and the pressure returned to normal when the patient awoke.

Another encouraging fact that was observed was that thirst increased ten to fifteen minutes after the infusion. The patients drank great quantities of water and their condition continued to improve. Appetite also returned and they ate with relish. As a rule the temperature during the first two days after recovery from shock was one to two degrees above normal and then gradually subsided.

Patients at the battalion mobile field hospitals could be followed for only three to seven days after which they were evacuated to divisional field hospitals, but in Tashkent they were followed for one to three months. In all cases, recovery was uneventful. Patients observed for prolonged periods of time showed no ill effects of any kind.

It was Dr. Pavlov who showed the way and it was Dr. Asratyan who followed the lead which resulted in the development of this new method of treating one of the most dangerous of all conditions: shock. It was Dr. Pavlov's belief that rest, particularly sleep, exerted important curative effects in profound disturbances of the nervous and blood-vessel systems. Dr. Asratyan confirmed Dr. Pavlov's concept experimentally by the treatment of traumatic shock through sleep induced by hypnotic drugs.

It was found, however, that sleep alone does not have a similar effect in all cases. Other healing measures have to be adopted in addition. The tone of the blood vessels must be raised, heart action has to be reinforced, tissue water-logging has to be eliminated, breathing has to be restored to normal and physiological processes have to be stimulated. This problem was solved by devising a solution which combined sedation with chemicals producing regulatory changes in the blood, vasomotor system and metabolism. This solution contains salines, bromides and hedonal. It is infused into the vein by the drip method, which means it is given slowly, drop by drop over a prolonged period of time. In the great majority of cases, Dr. Asratyan found that this method brought about complete recovery from shock.

XXVI

SOVIET STUDIES ON DEATH

FOR many years the phenomenon of death has attracted the attention of Soviet scientists. Among the first to become attracted to this study was Dr. S. J. Tchechulin, of the Chemico-Pharmaceutical Institute of the All-Russian Council for National Economy. Dr. Tchechulin carried out a series of very interesting experiments with a dog's head severed from its body and artificially supplied with perfusing liquid from a special apparatus. This experiment has shown that it is by no means essential for the organs to be directly connected with the body, even in the case of such a structure like the brain, with its exceptional sensitivity even to the impairment of the circulation.

In Dr. Tchechulin's experiments, the fundamental functions of the brain, especially the reflexes, remained quite distinct for from three and a half to four hours after the head had been severed. Several important conclusions are to be drawn from this fact. In the first place there is no difficulty in experimentally reproducing the mechanical conditions of the circulation, as normal circulation can easily be initiated by means of any suitable apparatus, capable of pumping blood into, and sucking it out of, the corresponding vessels, thus replacing the heart, provided the necessary temperature and pressure conditions are maintained.

In these experiments normal dog's blood was used for the perfusion liquid. In this manner the brain cells of the severed dog's head was supplied with the oxygen necessary for their normal function. The dog's head was apparently living although the rest of his body was dead. It had apparently been revived after having been severed from the rest of the body. The eyes had every appearance of life; the head responded to the slightest touch in typical lifelike movements. A caustic placed in the mouth was rejected. A piece of cheese placed on the tongue was swallowed. The head was actually living, though it had been severed from the body.

Speculations on the nature of death are to be found in the works of Ivan Pavlov, the greatest Russian physiologist who ever lived, as well as in the works of his pupils. Drs. A. A. Bogomolets and V. A. Negovski have advanced many new ideas on the nature of death. Basing their findings on experimental studies in the laboratory, as well as clinical experience in the hospitals, these Soviet doctors have made many interesting and important contributions to the study of death.

According to the latest Soviet researches, death is a condition which begins at the moment when the mathematically harmonious and coordinating activity existing among the vital centers of the organism is completely and finally disturbed. The essential cause of all death is this complete disruption of the coordinating vital activity, but the nature of death is twofold. There is (1) pathological (unnatural) and (2) physiological (natural) death.

Pathological death represents the greater problem because it is so infinite in number and variety. Fundamentally, however, pathologic death is of three kinds: mechanical death, chemical death and abnormal degenerative death. Mechanical death is brought about by a mechanical injury to the vital system, such as mechanical crushing of the organism. Chemical death is the result of a chemical reaction or set of chemical reactions within the organism, producing a condition incompatible with the coordinating activity of the vital centers. In such cases there is a substitution of the poison for the colloidal substance of the tissues. Thus, in the case of poisoning by arsenic, each molecule of the poison substitutes itself for at least six molecules of ionized water of the tissues. The tissues, thus deprived of their normal chemical constituency, are powerless to function normally, and if this condition is allowed to progress death will ensue. Abnormal degenerative death is brought about by a stimulated activity on the part of the conjunctive cells over the specialized cells. This is usually caused by some disease with its toxins or the introduction into the body of poisons which are the factors of stimulation.

In the majority of cases pathologic death is scarcely ever purely a mechanical or chemical death. More often it is a combination of both, or in some cases of all three. The primary variations are (1) Mechanico-chemical; (2) Chemico-mechanical; (3) Mechanico-degenerative; (4) Degenerative-chemical; (5) Chemico-degenerative; (6) Degenerative-mechanical and chemical disturbances. A mechanico-chemical death is death brought about by a mixed cause of mechanical and chemical disturbances of the vital activity of which the mechanical cause is the predominating factor. In the same way we may define the other five primary variations.

The secondary variations consist of (1) Mechanico-Chemico-degenerative; (2) Chemico-mechanico-degenerative; (3) Degenerative-chemico-mechanical, (4) Degenerative-mechanico-chemical; (5) Mechanico-degenerative-chemical; (6) Chemico-degenerative-mechanico-chemical. A mechanico-chemico-degenerative death is death brought on by a disturbance of the vital activity, partaking of every one of the three natures of pathologic death, and in the proportion in which the mechanical predominates over the chemical, which in turn, predominates over the degenerative cause. The remaining five variations may be similarly defined.

Pathologic death, which is so varied, may thus be conveniently classified. It is by far the more common of the two, and the majority of living organisms come to the death pathologically. While there may be some faint hope of eradicating physiologic death, pathologic death can never be effectively resisted by man.

Physiologic, or natural death, is the incidental result of cellular differentiation. Weismann's views on the advent of physiological death are of significance:

"1. Natural death occurs only among the multicellular beings: it is not found among unicellular organisms. The process of encystment in the latter is by no means comparable with death.

"2. Natural death first appears among the lowest heteroplastid metazoa in the limitation of all cells collecting to one generation, and of the somatic or body cells proper to a restricted period; the somatic cells afterward in the higher metazoa come to last several and even many generations, and life was lengthened to a corresponding degree.

"3. This limitation went hand in hand with a differentiation of the cells of the organism into reproductive and somatic cells, in accordance with the principle of the division of labor. This differentiation took place by the operation of natural selection.

"4. The fundamental biogenetic law only applies to the multicellular being but it does not apply to the unicellular forms of life. This depends, on the other hand, upon the mode of reproduction by fission which obtains among monoplastids (unicellular organisms), and, on the other, upon the necessity induced by sexual reproduction for the maintenance of the unicellular stage in the development of the polyplastids (multicellular organisms).

"5. Death itself, and the longer or shorter duration of life, both depend solely upon adaptation. Death is not an essential attribute of living matter; it is not necessarily associated with reproduction, nor is it a necessary consequence of it."

Exactly what is the process of physiological dying in a highly specialized individual? There are several ways in which this process may be viewed. There begins, from the day of birth of the complex organism, a struggle between the primitive and specialized cells, and this continues throughout life. Disease, poisons, or tissue tramata may cause an overactivity of the primitive element (conjunctive cells) and hasten death, which in such a case would be pathological. On the other hand, if there is an absence of abnormal excitement of the conjuctive cells and they continue to bring triumph over the specialized cells in a normal manner, physiologic death will result.

This activity of the primitive element tends to bring all back to a primitive condition, where each cell was sufficient unto itself. But the highly specialized organism is one where everything is coordinated and this leveling process is fatal. The conjunctive cells replacing the highly specialized ones are in no way capable of carrying out the highly organized and coordinating activity, and finally, there occurs a complete disturbance of the vital activity, and naturally death is the result.

This phenomenon of displacement of specialized cells by primitive ones occurs everywhere in the tissues—and the relation that these tissues bear to the vital activity affects the maintenance of life in a definite proportion. The fatty degeneration of the heart is of greater concern than fatty degeneration elsewhere in the body. Primitive cells (the osteoclasts) multiply around the osseous laminae, whence they draw the pith of the bony substance. The muscles undergo the same degeneration, being invaded by the primitive protoplasm (the sarcoplasm).

What is the normal duration of time consumed in the final culmination of the triumph of the primitive over the specialized element? Buffon claimed that the normal duration of time was six to seven times that of the period of growth, but he erroneously maintained that fourteen was the age at which the growth terminated. Elourens properly fixed the age at which the process of growth comes to an end at twenty, at which age the bones have ceased their growth. Thus, the normal span of life is from 120 to 140 years.

We may now arrive at a definition of physiologic death from the viewpoint of the struggle between the primitive and specialized elements in the body of a highly specialized organism; physiologic death is the final culmination of the triumph (stimulated in their process by any cause whatever) of the conjunctive cells over the specialized cells, to bring about, by their unstimulated degenerative invasion of the vital organism, a complete disturbance of the mathematically harmonious and coordinating activity existing among them. Any deviation from this at once falls into the province of pathologic death.

Biological chemistry offers a supplementary explanation of the process of physiologic death. This process is one of dea-quifications by aggregation. This takes place in the aging of all organic colloids, and is claimed to be the one which changed the organism from its embryo stage to senility and which finally ends in death. In the human species this process extrudes H_2O and defines the process of life from birth to natural death. Old age, expressed in terms of the biochemistry of senile degeneration, is a certain stage of deaquification of the propoplasm of the tissues. This process of deaquification may be represented by the following equations:

$$Pm\ (OH\ H)\ N\ No.\ Pm\ (OH\ H)\ N\ No.\ N\ H_2O.$$
$$2\ Pm\ (OH\ H)\ N\ No.\ 2\ Pm\ (OH\ H)\ N-N\ H_2O.$$

$Pm\ (OH\ H)\ N$ represents the colloidal protoplasm of the human tissues, and Pm represents the protoplasm.

Biological chemistry has brought down the definition of physiologic death to a formula. The more interesting problem would be to discover a formula or a series of formulae to represent the vital process known as life.

At the present time studies on the causes of death are being carried out at various medical centers in the Soviet Union by Drs. I. R. Petrov, V. A. Negovski, A. D. Speranski, Prawdicz-Neminski and others. They are studying biochemical and biophysical phenomena connected with the death of the organism and methods that may be employed to reverse the process of dying in the early stages. A thorough understanding of death and its mechanism has already yielded practical results in many cases of death caused by accident and disease. The revival of the dying organism is now an accomplished fact in many instances, thanks to the latest discoveries of Dr. V. A. Negovski.

XXVII

INJECTING BLOOD INTO THE HEART

THE Red Army soldier had sustained a shell splinter wound of the neck. The splinter was removed seventeen days later. A second operation was performed several weeks afterward to repair the injury to a large blood vessel which the splinter had inflicted. The blood vessel was weakened and bulged dangerously. It looked as if it would rupture any moment, and it was during the operation that it did rupture. Despite all efforts to arrest it, the blood continued to flow in a vigorous, pulsating stream. A minute later the pupils became widely dilated, the reaction to lights disappeared, the eyeballs became soft, and deadly pallor and marked chilling of the body occurred. The breathing stopped, the pulse could not be felt, the heart sounds could not be heard.

The surgeon, Dr. B. I. Iokhveds immediately realized that the patient was dying and that energetic efforts were immediately required to save his life. A long needle was inserted into the fourth interspace in the chest, somewhat to the left of the breastbone margin. After a few seconds, irregular movements were transmitted to the needle. Then an apparatus filled with physiologic saline solution was connected with the needle inserted into the heart. During all that time the heart contractions were very weak, the tension of the eyeballs diminished, and breathing and pulse could not be detected.

Five hundred cubic centimeters of physiologic salt solution were injected. Three or four minutes after the injection was started, the pulsation of the heart grew stronger. The pulse reached 100 beats per minute, and shallow, irregular breathing was resumed. The intracardiac needle became obstructed and was withdrawn. A second needle was inserted further to the left. At that moment, the pulse disappeared again and the blood stopped flowing from the exposed vein. Breathing stopped and only a faint thrust of the needle could be felt. Three hundred c.c. of whole blood were then transfused into the heart followed by 50 c.c. of physiologic saline solution. During the transfusion, there was a pronounced pulsation of the needle. The pulse was fuller and rhythmic. The breathing was deep and regular. The pupils resumed their normal size and began to react to light. The man was out of danger. He was brought back to the land of the living.

Injections into the heart of adrenalin have been used for many years to restore the heart to activity after it had ceased to beat. In 1935 Dr. Lian reported satisfactory results from the injection of ouabain into the heart in cases of heart failure. Following this, Russian surgeons became very much interested in intracardiac injections and experimented on animals by injecting various substances into the heart to get it beating again. Lately, Dr. B. I. Iokhveds used saline solution and blood to inject into the heart to revive its activity.

Dr. Iokhveds is of the opinion that application of massage to the heart externally and the injection of adrenalin in severe cases is not enough, because there is a lack of supply of blood to the heart. The heart, even when revived, will continue to work in a vacuum, and after a few seconds or minutes will stop again. It was for this reason that Dr. Iokhveds decided to adopt more physiologic methods by increasing the contents of the cavities of the heart. It is a well-known fact that an increase in the contents is an adequate impulse to start contraction, as long as the heart is capable of responding to stimulation.

In the case cited, injection of blood and salt solution into the left ventricle of the heart rather than the right was indicated for a definite reason. Insufficient contracting force of the recently revived heart and the pressure behind the injected solution would be insufficient to overcome the resistance provided by the capillary network in the lungs and only a very small amount would reach the left side of the heart. By injecting these solutions directly into the left cavity of the heart, even the first and comparatively weak contractions of the heart reestablish the blood supply to the vitally important brain centers, thus providing an anti-shock effect.

Says Dr. Iokhveds: "Intracardiac transfusions of blood, and possibly other substances, employing the right as well as the left ventricles, are means which in combination with other standard methods of therapy could prove useful to every physician in the fight for the revival of men dying from shock and collapse due to various causes."

It is quite apparent that injections into the heart must be begun almost immediately after the heart has ceased to beat. Dr. Iokhveds begins from eight to ten seconds after clinical death has appeared. In some cases it is possible to get good results even after two to six minutes. In all cases quick action is essential.

Another recent advance in the use of blood as a life-saving measure was the introduction of auto-blood-transfusion or blood replacement. It is used in cases where profuse internal bleeding takes place through the rupture of an important artery. In these cases there is no preliminary typing or other blood examination. It is simply a process of taking the escaped blood and putting it back into the patient's veins. This has now become a common practice in the Soviet Union.

Reanimation of the heart is one of the greatest contributions of surgery to the preservation of human life. While there is even the slightest flicker of life there is hope, and many persons now living owe their lives to surgeons who persisted in attempting to get the heart to start beating again.

XXVIII

THE HEALTH VALUE OF AIR

SOVIET scientists have not been content to explore only along known and familiar lines. One of their greatest gifts is exploring the unknown, venturing along new and unfamiliar paths, probing into places that are still virgin territory. One of these explorers of the unknown is Dr. N. G. Cholodny.

One of the things that always puzzled Dr. Cholodny was why sick people always derived great benefit when they went to the country and began filling their lungs with country air. Why does health come back to those broken in body when they go to the mountains and breathe pure mountain air? Why is the air of a pine forest so invigorating?

All these facts are known to most of us, but very few of us ever thought of trying to uncover the reason for this fact. Dr. Cholodny, however, is a man of vast curiosity and, after researches of three years, announced that certain substances in nature's unpolluted air are essential to human health. There are several varieties of these substances and among them are vitamins and hormones as well as biochemicals that eliminate bacteria which cause disease. Dr. Cholodny is a biochemist and a member of the Soviet Academy of Sciences.

It is these substances, believes Dr. Cholodny, these atmospheric particles which affect cures when worn-out, ill people begin to breathe pure country air or mountain air. This air is a veritable tonic, a health-giving tonic of real curative value.

Dr. Cholodny is a scientist of world-wide reputation. His native Ukraine was invaded by the Germans and he was driven from his laboratory. He continued his researches in the Armenian Soviet Republic. Here in 1943 he discovered that growing plants—especially sprouting seeds, leaves, pine needles, flowers and fruits—give off into the air a very small but measurable quantity of complex chemicals. It is these chemicals, Cholodny found, that have the power of stimulating man and animals.

The quantity of these substances in the air is rather small, not enough to supply body-building or energy-producing nourishment. But since the material is readily absorbed in our lungs, it has been found to exert a definite effect on the germs causing tuberculosis.

In one of his reports Dr. Cholodny has said: "It may prove that among other causes responsible for lung tuberculosis, this disease is caused also by a peculiar kind of vitamin deficiency of the lungs, related to the lack of life-stimulating substances in the air of our cities."

These ideas and speculations of Dr. Cholodny are not merely those of one man. They have been confirmed by others. E. H. Lucas and R. W. Lewis, American biochemists, associated with the Michigan State College of Agriculture and Applied Science, have ascertained that leaves, fruits and other plant parts contain powerful germ-killers like penicillin. They isolated such substances in honeysuckle, peony, Scotch thistle, mountain ash and blueberry.

Dr. Cholodny's researches along this line have brought to light two remarkable facts. The first is that the potent "herbal chemicals" not only exist inside growing plants, but some at least are given off into the air. The second is that the germ-killing substances are accompanied in the air by chemicals of far greater influence, those which resemble vitamins and hormones in their effects and actions.

So little of these substances are actually required for health that a sufficient amount exists in the air to exert a favorable effect. Dr. Cholodny has demonstrated that the air contains at least one one-millionth part of active substances. Since an adult breathes 100 to 140 ounces of air per day— more than our intake of food—the lungs would get three to four milligrams of "atmospheric vitamins." It has been estimated that this quantity is just about the weight of ordinary vitamins we require in our daily food.

It has been known for many years now that when even minute amounts of vitamins are missing from our daily intake we are in time stricken by such diseases like pellagra, scurvy and beri-beri. These ailments are cured by supplying the proper vitamins.

In a like manner these researches by Dr. Cholodny raise the question whether many other diseases may be caused by breathing vitamin-deficient air. This thought is shared by many scientists. Dr. Clarence A. Mills has said: "Fortunately for the medical profession, climatic therapy offers greatest benefits for those very diseases in which other forms of treatment have been least helpful."

One of the facts brought to light by climatology is that winter sharply lowers our resistance to respiratory and other ailments. Sexual fertility is decreased. When spring comes there is something in the very air that brings about an improvement and we are less prone to disease. Why?

Dr. Cholodny offers the following explanation. The springtime melting of snow and covering of the earth with new growing plants, fills the air with stimulating biochemicals. Dr. Cholodny has ascertained that dry air contains far more of these active substances than moist air. Tropical rain and jungle mist remove these materials rapidly. Also, it has been found that inhaling too much of these atmospheric vitamins, or of certain kinds, may be harmful.

"This is especially true," says Dr. Cholodny, "of substances evolved by flowers. In the interpretation here advanced, these phenomenona may well be compared with hypvitaminosis."

Dr. Cholodny's discoveries are of the greatest importance.

Some years ago the discovery of vitamins in foods revolutionized nutrition and medicine and helped solve the problem of certain diseases which could not be cured by medicine and surgery but which could be cured by eating the proper foods. The same may be true of Dr. Cholodny's discoveries. It is possible that these vital biochemicals in the air may be found to exert curative effects on such diseases like arthritis, tuberculosis, influenza and other ailments about which not too much is known at the present time.

The pollution of city air with smoke and other substances may destroy these biochemicals and thus promote disease. Atmospheric studies by health authorities are very important in ascertaining just how these pollutions of the atmosphere affect our health. Industrial hygiene is rapidly finding out that the air we breathe is as important to maintaining health as the food we eat.

The interest in the air as a source of health has been claiming the attention of medicine for more than 2,000 years. Hippocrates was interested in the air, what it contained and how it affected health. The search for these substances went on for many years, and it is only within the past several decades that physicists and chemists have learned that the atmosphere contains many important gases and other chemical substances which are absolutely necessary to maintain life and also to maintain health.

Says Dr. Cholodny: "The salutary effects on the air of woods, of prairies, and of vast areas overgrown by a diversified and abundant vegetation has been known long since. This fact, which until recently has defied satisfactory explanation, may easily be understood if we are to assume that some phytogenic substances of the atmosphere are necessary for our organism, as accessory food factors or vitamins."

Dr. Cholodny's work has been among the pioneer efforts along this line. Research is going forward on the biochemicals of the atmosphere and how they affect our health. It is possible that biochemists may soon analyze and ascertain just what these chemicals are. The next step may be to make them artificially and increase their abundance in places where they are scarce.

When this is accomplished we may be able to bring mountain air and pure country air into our bedrooms by means of vaporizers which will instill these chemicals into the air of our immediate surroundings. There is no doubt that Dr. Cholodny's researches on the mysterious biochemicals in the air and how they influence our well-being will prove one of the great advances of modern medicine.

XXIX

METHODS OF TREATING FROSTBITE

LIVING in a country where temperatures drop to many degrees below zero, Soviet medical men have been especially interested in the problems of frostbite. Some of the most recent methods of combating this condition were evolved in the Soviet Union. Among the most thorough investigators of frostbite is Dr. S. S. Girgolav, who has been invesigating frostbite since 1934. At first these investigations were purely experimental, but during the war with Finland, and later the war with Germany, much of value was learned from a clinical point of view.

A number of investigations conducted by Dr. Ariev resulted in the discovery of new facts at variance with commonly accepted views regarding frostbite. Most people believed that slow warming of the body was indicated in frostbite. Drs. Ariev, Shainis and Moldavanov proved that rapid warming of frostbite is better and should be used in treating frostbitten parts of the body.

Another fallacy which has prevailed up till now was that the frozen parts of the body, such as the nose, ears, fingers and toes, are unusually fragile. That has been proved to be erroneous. They are no more fragile when cold than they are when warm.

Studies on the effect of cold on the human body has demonstrated that warm clothing, which does not interfere with circulation, is a very good protection against frostbite. Also essential are dry footwear and a diet rich in fats and carbohydrates. Soviet doctors have found that the healthy skin of a warmly dressed, physically fit person offers the best protection against frostbite.

Soviet authorities divide frostbite into four instead of three types. First degree frostbite involves only the skin. Involvement of the superficial layers under the skin is second degree frostbite, while third degree involves the upper muscular layers. Fourth degree involves the deep muscles and the bones.

Dr. D. I. Panchenko studied the effects of frostbite on the nervous system and came forth with some very interesting and important facts. He found that frostbite may be followed by retrograde degeneration of the peripheral nerves, preceded by irritation of and damage to the cells. It also may produce harmful changes in the spinal cord. Another interesting fact that Dr. Panchenko discovered was that frostbite, because of its effect on the nervous system, produces a heightened susceptibility and frequent recurrence of infection. It was also found that such conditions as obliterative endarteritis, a disease of the blood vessels, and spontaneous gangrene may follow severe cases of frostbite in which damage has been done to the blood vessels.

The treatment of frostbite has claimed the attention of Soviet doctors within recent years. The severe winter of 1941-42 brought them face to face with the problem of finding means of preventing frostbite among the troops. At that time great importance was attached to the use of various greases and ointments. The troops were advised to use ointments not only on the chin, nose and ears, but also to saturate the foot cloths.

Dr. F. G. Krotkov became very much interested in the treatment of frostbite. He conducted experiments with various ointments in Leningrad and showed that the vascular reaction of the skin is altered very slightly with any of the ointments. Temperature curves of the extremities did not vary from the controls. Most of the men undergoing the tests felt no effects from the use of the ointments. Seventy-five per cent of them complained of an unpleasant sticky sensation. As a result of these experiments the following conclusions were drawn:

1. Because of the transitory effect on the skin, use of ointments is advisable only during a brief stay indoors.

2. Not one of the tested ointments should be recommended for long expeditions during cold weather.

3. Soap and water remove the sticky ointment from the skin with difficulty.

4. Prolonged application of the ointments interfere with metabolism of the skin by obstructing the pores. Use of any grease on the feet predisposes them to maceration.

A medical commission was appointed by the Director of Medical Services of the Leningrad front. After much experimentation they arrived at the conclusion that the kind of base and the moisture content determine the actual value of the ointment. This commission recommended an ointment consisting of 20 gms. of camphor, 5 gms. of bees' wax, and 80 gms. of anhydrous petrolatum. This ointment contains no irritants of any kind.

When tested on a large scale in the late war, this ointment did not produce any remarkable results. Men complained that the ointment produced "burning" and "cutting" of the skin and after one application refused to try it again. Further tests with this ointment showed that frostbite was not prevented by using it.

Consequently, as a result of many tests, the Surgical Section of the Scientific Medical Council adopted the following resolution: "Because of the detrimental tendency to employ protective ointments at the front, the medical officers must be given orders to restrict the use of greases and ointments to the exposed parts of the body. The use of greases or ointments for rubbing in to the feet and for saturating the footcloths is to be categorically prohibited."

After more study and investigation the committee of the

Scientific Medical Council suggested that pure petrolatum replace all the ointments for the prevention of frostbite since petrolatum contains no skin irritants, is free from moisture, may be applied freely to exposed parts of the body, and is easily removed with soap and warm water.

The experience of the late war supported these findings and proved that properly fitted shoes, dry socks and foot-cloths, insoles made of felt, cloth or straw, and sufficiently roomy and dry clothing are the most adequate means of combating frostbite. Particularly, attention has to be paid to the hygiene of the feet. The footcloths should be changed frequently, and the foot wear should be kept dry and in good condition.

The effects of cold on the body were studied by Drs. Frenkel, S. T. Pavlov and Bykov and many interesting facts were brought to light. Due to the poor heat-conductivity of human tissues, the effect of cold is in direct proportion to the length of exposure. Time, therefore, plays a very important role in chilling. It is well known that the brief action of cold, as employed in local anesthesia, is tolerated without ill effect. If the action is prolonged, the circulation is interfered with and damage to the tissues results.

Theories of frostbite which are based on the conception that water within the cells turns into ice are without foundation. It is not necessary that the water within the cell turn to ice to bring about death of the cell. Cell damage takes place even when the water in the cell is fluid.

Another popular fallacy which has been exploded by the Soviet doctors in their studies on frostbite is that the use of snow or ice water to warm the frozen part is of no value; in fact, it is a harmful procedure. The use of snow or ice water enhances chilling and aggravates the condition. The warming should be done by the use of warm water, not hot water. The warming should be done rather quickly. There is no harm in rapid warming.

METHODS OF TREATING FROSTBITE   199

Many interesting facts about bodily physiology have come to light as the result of these frostbite studies. Thus, one of these investigations has revealed a reflex somatic disturbance following localized damage. Further research along this line is called for. There are still other problems connected with frostbite that require research, and there is no doubt that more interesting facts will be forthcoming in the near future.

XXX

DENTAL HEALTH

THE foremost investigator on dental health in the Soviet Union is Dr. I. Lukomski, who has studied the possibilities of fluorine in improving and maintaining oral hygiene.

For many years Dr. Lukomski has been immersed in the study of methods of preventing tooth decay. His investigations may be considered as being divided into two phases. The first phase, a laboratory study in which he subjected his ideas to rigid experimental tests, and second, a clinical phase in which he studied the effects of these discoveries on patients.

In his laboratory Dr. Lukomski has conducted many interesting experiments in which he demonstrated that the application of varying concentrations of sodium fluoride solutions to the tooth structure makes for a stable combination between the fluoride and the dental tissues. He has also found that there is a marked alteration in the permeability of dental tissues that have been exposed to concentrated fluoride solutions. Bacteriological studies have revealed that fluoride solutions have an unfavorable effect on germ life.

As a result of his laboratory work Dr. Lukomski has discovered two primary clinical uses for fluorine. The first of these is the internal administration of sodium fluoride for the treatment of pyorrhea. In the treatment of pyorrhea he uses a one per cent solution of sodium fluoride at the rate of three drops three times a day for approximately three weeks. The reason for using sodium fluoride is that it stimulates recalcification of the area around the teeth and possibly inhibits a thyroid factor that may bear a causative relationship to the condition.

Dr. Lukomski has found fluorine therapy of particular value in cases that are characterized by the presence of gingivitis and progressive atrophy of the dental tissues. More than five hundred cases were treated with this chemical and the treatment has been shown to be effective especially in those cases where there has been only mild or moderate lessening of the teeth. It has been found that in these instances the teeth tend to become firm, the chewing efficiency of the patient is increased, inflammation disappears and bleeding of the gums stops.

The second form of treatment advocated by Dr. Lukomski is local in nature. Dr. Lukomski has reasoned that since fluoride has a great affinity for calcium phosphates, locally applied fluoride forms a chemical union with the dentin. This means that fluoride is of value in the treatment of hypersensitive dentin such as may be encountered when cavities exist. Under these conditions sodium fluoride is applied in the form of a paste containing equal parts of white clay and glycerine. The paste is applied to the affected area and burnished for periods of five minutes. In most of the cases one treatment is sufficient. The more serious cases may require several such treatments. To date over 5,000 cases have been treated successfully in this manner.

Dr. Lukomski has also used sodium fluoride in the recalcification of softened dentin in over 600 cases. A paste of .7 per cent sodium fluoride is sealed on the floor of the cavity. This has been found to arrest further development of caries. Gangrenous root canals have also yielded nicely to the treatment with sodium fluoride. It has been observed that following such treatment there is a reduction in the number of acid-forming bacteria in the area. In many cases treated it has been ascertained that the dentin hardens and that further cavity formation in the teeth are arrested permanently. Also germ life inimical to the teeth are greatly reduced in number.

Another interesting fact that Dr. Lukomski has discovered in his work with sodium fluoride is that fluoride therapy may be indicated in the implantation, replantation and transplantation of teeth. These methods have fallen into disuse mainly because the teeth so treated usually undergo considerable alteration due to resorption of minerals. Since fluoride-treated tooth structures have been demonstrated to be harder and less permeable, it seems reasonable to believe that the immersion of the teeth in fluoride solutions prior to operation might prevent this difficulty. However, much research along this line is indicated.

XXXI

REBUILDING MEN'S HOPES

THE greatest genito-urinary surgeon in the Soviet Union is Dr. A. P. Frumkin, who is also the chief genito-urinary surgeon of the Red Army. His accomplishments in the way of plastic surgery in reconstructing man's reproductive organs destroyed by war or accident are among the miracles of modern surgery. Dr. Frumkin is not the first surgeon to graft new male sex organs, but he is certainly the first to apply it on a great scale and he has been more successful than anyone else.

The use of new and highly destructive weapons in war resulted in a large number of wounds which were comparatively unknown in earlier wars. The rapid fire of automatic weapons and mine and bomb explosions with their spray of fragments have resulted in numerous injuries and often in the destruction of whole organs.

It was not at all surprising that the complete loss of the external reproductive organs was a rather frequent occurrence during the late war. The explosion of a mine at close range often led to the destruction of the male genital organs.

"I have seen men at the front, carried off the battlefield. They plead for death. They do not want to live," Dr. Frumkin said. "My first job is always to convince the wounded that there is hope.

"Two years ago, three years ago, I had little faith in myself. Now I can speak concretely of results. I can show them pictures. I can even let them speak to men who have been restored fully—both mentally and physically.

203

"All the skills of modern plastic surgery must be mobilized to reconstruct the missing genital organ. The surgeon must not only recreate the missing penis but restore its function as well. The last consideration is of paramount importance where one or both testes are preserved. Moreover, there have been a number of cases in which the sexual impulse persisted for a long time after the loss of both testes in which the sexual act was possible when the penis was present."

Dr. Frumkin is considerate and patient with each new patient who comes to him for treatment. The entire process is explained to the man at length and in simple, easily understood terms. He is brought into contact with other patients who are recovering or have recovered. The operation must be done carefully and precisely. Reconstruction of the external genitalia after a traumatic loss is performed as a rule in four stages.

The operation is one in which skill and ingenuity enter. In simple terms Dr. Frumkin makes a new organ from the cartilaginous portions of the eighth and ninth ribs (the cartilaginous portions being the softer and more pliable material found in the ribs). This remains in close contact with its original location while a tube is formed inside the flap of skin.

After about a month the top of the future organ is severed from its original position and transferred to the abdomen. The entire series of operations takes from six to ninth months, for the operation is done by careful stages and healing must be complete before the next step can be undertaken.

As stated before, the entire process consists of four major stages which are as follows:

1. Formation of an abdominal skin tube into which rib cartilage is inserted.

2. Transfer of the near pedicle of the tube and implantation of the cartilage into the remnants of the cavernous bodies.

3. Division of the far end of the tube and formation of the penis.

4. Reconstruction of the urethral canal.

Through these four stages an organ is reconstructed which not only corrects the cosmetic defect but assumes the normal sexual function as well. The latter depends upon some remaining parts of the cavernous bodies. Their tumefaction under the influence of sexual impulses moves the cartilaginous portion of the penis upward and forward so that sexual relations are possible. Normal sexual activity is possible with the new organ.

Dr. Frumkin has performed several hundred of these operations up to this date, all of which have been successful. "My patients have been happily married, and they have produced normal offspring," Dr. Frumkin declares. "Quentin Reynolds said there would be a lot of postwar babies named Frumkin."

Dr. Frumkin is now occupied with the problem of testicular grafting to correct the most serious cases in which there has been a loss of the testes. He has now arrived at a stage in his work where the grafting of testicles is practical and possible. This makes success in the reconstruction of new male sex organs complete.

One of his most spectacular cases was one in which he grafted the right testicle with good results. The man was an officer who had been wounded in a mine explosion which resulted in a loss of both testicles. He was sent to Botkin Hospital where he came under the care of Dr. Frumkin. He was treated for shock and given general treatment to build up his strength.

Within a month the loss of the testicles began to have their effects on this officer. His body began to take on fat, his voice became shrill and piping; his hair stopped growing; in other words he was turning into a eunuch, a man without a sex.

Dr. Frumkin then decided that the only operation that

would be of any value was one in which the testicles could be transplanted into the body of this officer. The patient was very eager for this operation.

The object was now to get the testicles with which to perform the transplant. The Moscow hospitals were put on the alert; when a young man of the same blood group as the officer was fatally injured in a street car accident, he was rushed to Botkin Hospital, and as soon as he died Dr. Frumkin operated. He removed the right testicle along with its blood vessels and other attachments. This was immediately transplanted under the skin of the officer's right thigh about eight inches below the hip bone. Then he sewed the arteries to the femoral artery and the vein to the femoral vein, and thus a complete blood vessel connection with the host's body was established.

All that Dr. Frumkin could now do was to wait and see what would happen. Within a period of four months the new testicle had established the proper physiological connections in the officer's body. It had become acclimatized; it was viable and was in intimate connection with the blood vessels and the testicle was normal and functioning.

In time the officer lost his surplus fat; his hair began to grow normally again; his voice became masculine in pitch and timbre. The officer, who had previously lost interest in women, was now experiencing a reawakened interest in the opposite sex.

There is still another operation to perform before Dr. Frumkin can be satisfied and that is transferring the testicle from the officer's thigh into its proper place in the scrotum. "This portion of the operation will be less difficult than what has already been accomplished," Dr. Frumkin states.

When this final stage of the operation has been accomplished the officer will be a stage nearer sexual normality than before. Upon its completion he will be able to function more or less normally as a husband, although he will be sterile and not able to beget children.

"At this stage of my experiment, it is premature to call this anything but the purest kind of experiment—I have not gone so far as to consider making a connection with the spermatic cord." Should Dr. Frumkin be able to make a connection with the spermatic cord the officer will then be able to have children. But that is something for the future to decide.

The work of Dr. Frumkin is among the most important that has come out of the U.S.S.R. It restores life, hope and manhood to men who have been horribly mutilated and left without hope. Before Dr. Frumkin perfected his operations many such men committed suicide rather than face life without the hope of ever being normal in the way they had a right to be. Other surgeons are now following the technique as laid out by Dr. Frumkin, and the benefits of his operation are now available all over the world.

XXXII

ACCOMPLISHMENTS OF SOVIET NEUROSURGEONS

NEUROSURGERY has developed by leaps and bounds in the Soviet Union within the past ten years. Much of great value was learned during the late war; but even before that experimental studies had been carried out on animals by such men as Dr. V. N. Shamov and Dr. Anokhin. The latter started experimental studies on dogs with canine nerves at the Neurophysiological Laboratory of the All-Union Institute of Experimental Medicine. He isolated a nerve, cut sections of it, and filled the defects with the nerve of another dog, which had been immersed in a 10-15 per cent solution of formalin for ten to fifteen days. It was found that this formalinized nerve sector acted as a bridge of dead tissue over which the regenerating central nerve sector reached the outer section of the other nerve.

These were the beginnings. Other and more extensive experiments were performed using formalinized canine nerves to overcome nerve defects. The Institute of Experimental Medicine reported encouraging results along this line as did other clinics. It was then that Dr. Ignatov of the Institute of Experimental Medicine decided to use formalinized human nerves taken from corpses to overcome nerve defects in human beings. He used a nerve similar to the defective nerve so that both human nerves would have the same diameter.

It was during the Finnish War that Soviet neurosurgeons had the first great opportunity to use transplanted nerves. During this war there were thirteen cases of so great severity of nerve damage that direct contact of the severed nerves was impossible. It was in these cases that new nerves were used, transplanted from others to overcome the defects. The size of the implanted nerve varied with the size of the defect. One case was that in which the sciatic, the largest nerve in the body, was severed, and a transplant was made with the sciatic nerve taken from a corpse. The final results were perfect. Other damaged nerves that were repaired were the median, radial and ulnar nerves. All nerves were restored to good function.

This newly devised method of formalinized nerve implantation has the advantage of reestablishing function in cases in which the injury to the nerve is so extensive that the two ends cannot be reunited. For that reason new nerve tissue has to be used.

Another factor that the Soviet nerve surgeons have learned to take into consideration is that early treatment is required in order to get the best results. Drs. Babitski, Bakulev, Lebedenko, Neklepaeva and Geimanovich after a great deal of laboratory and clinical experience arrived at the following conclusions:

1. The nervous system controls the course of the pathologic processes not only in the injured nerve but also in the infected wounds.

2. Early elimination of harmful stimuli caused by the nerve injuries exerts a favorable influence on regeneration and restoration of the nerve function and on the healing of wounds.

3. For completely severed nerves early interference provides an opportunity to approximate the cut ends and thereby to avoid transplantation.

Dr. M. L. Borovski and Dr. B. S. Doinikov, working in Dr. Speransky's laboratory, have unveiled many important facts regarding nerve injuries which have been used in treatment with remarkably good results. The following conclusions were arrived at after much experimentation and have influenced nerve surgeons throughout the world.

1. The distant end of the injured nerve is not only viable but still united indirectly with the body.

2. In certain forms of injury the condition of the distal severed nerve ending determines the development of some abnormal processes.

3. By repairing this end of the nerve the pathologic process is halted and improvement results.

Various nerve operations have been devised and widely used in the Soviet Union to abolish pain. Operations on the spinal cord for the relief of pain are now more commonly performed in serious ailments, as are operations for facial neuralgia. Even a radical operation in which a great deal of nervous tissue is removed is often performed with the utmost safety and without any danger from loss of muscle action of the face and tongue, which previously was a complication most feared.

Painful conditions of internal organs are often alleviated by certain nerve operations which Soviet neurosurgeons perform with utmost skill and confidence. An operation for dividing the presacral nerve has been yielding very good results for the relief of intractible pelvic pain in women.

The treatment of spastic paralysis, particularly when caused by gun-shot wounds, by certain nerve operations has been developed to a high stage of perfection in the U.S.S.R. By destroying certain bits of nerve tissue which cause this type of paralysis a great improvement in the condition becomes apparent in a short time.

Nerve surgery of the blood vessels also is finding wide application in the treatment of contraction of large blood vessels which ultimately may result in gangrene. Many remarkable cases have been reported in which nerve surgery of this kind has resulted in the saving of limbs destined for atrophy and disuse.

A great deal of interesting work has been done by Soviet nerve surgeons on that part of the nervous system known as the sympathetic nervous system, which controls all inner bodily activities, particularly the glands of internal secretion. At times there is a speeding up of inner bodily activity by overactive nerves which results in many abnormal conditions.

Such diseases as diabetes, hyperthyroidism, stomach ulcers and asthenia are the results of disturbances of the sympathetic nervous system. Rather simple nerve operations have been devised in which certain delicate nerves enervating these glands of internal secretion are destroyed. This results in a relief of the high tension within the body and a decided improvement in the over-all condition.

This operation is simple and entirely free from danger and the results following it are most remarkable. The day following the operation the patient notices a lessening of consciousness of his heart. Nervous tension is gone. There is a decrease in perspiration and warming of the skin.

As time goes on other benefits are noticeable. The most agreeable of these is the permanent emotional improvement in those patients who, before the operation, were irritable, unstable and unbearable. But this is only one of the benefits. Persistent headache is relieved; also relieved are annoying indigestion, gaseous eructions and other stomach discomforts.

This operation has been employed in more serious derangement of the sympathetic nervous system, such as stomach ulcers, diabetes and even epilepsy. Surgeons have noted that excessive activity of the thyroid is so much benefited by this simple operation that the more serious operation of removing part of the thyroid is sometimes avoided.

Perhaps the most dramatic results have been in the improvement in cases of stomach ulcers. In many cases the nerve operation is sufficient in curing the ulcer without resorting to the more serious and difficult operation of operating on the stomach itself.

Epilepsy of certain kinds are helped permanently by destroying a few fine strands of nerve tissue. In certain types of high blood pressure, this operation has been of benefit in arresting the disease and sometimes even actually curing it. There are also certain types of diabetes in which good results are obtained when the nervous link to the adrenal glands are destroyed.

Nerve surgery is going on apace in the U.S.S.R. Daily, new methods are being discovered for the treatment of serious nerve injuries as well as nerve diseases. Diseases which were previously regarded as hopeless and beyond cure are now being alleviated and in many cases even cured. The work of Dr. Speransky in evaluating the role of the nervous system in health and disease has served as a wonderful stimulus to all nerve surgeons who have worked with him in his laboratories and clinics, or those who are acquainted with his discoveries.

XXXIII

A GREAT RESEARCH INSTITUTE

A VERY familiar set of initials which you will encounter countless times in Soviet medical literature are V.I.E.M. This is the abbreviation of the Marxim Gorki All-Union Institute of Experimental Medicine in Moscow. This Institute was organized on October 15, 1932, to replace the old Institute of Experimental Medicine, which was the only large research institute in Czarist Russia. The original Institute was founded in St. Petersburg in 1890, and Pasteur and Koch collaborated in establishing it. It had many famous names connected with it, among them, Ivan Pavlov, of conditioned reflex fame, Vinogradsky, the bacteriologist, Uskov, the anatomist.

The original Institute of Experimental Medicine was the foremost medical research center in old Russia. It became the gathering place of physicians who wished to further their medical knowledge and to undertake original medical research. Metchnikov and Virchow were frequent visitors to the Institute. In 1900 it was visited by a group of American medical men who studied its organization in preparation for the foundation of the Rockefeller Institute for Medical Research.

The leading light of the old Institute was, of course, Ivan Pavlov, one of the world's greatest physiologists. He attracted many brilliant medical men who later rose to great fame in their own right. Among these we may mention Konstantin M. Bykov, who showed the influence of the brain on the functions of the various internal organs, and Alexei D.

213

Speransky, who studied the role of the nervous system in various abnormal conditions of the body and who announced a new theory of medicine based on these very important facts.

Because of the fact that Maxim Gorki had always been interested in the affairs of the Institute, the old Institute was reorganized in 1932 by decree of the Council of People's Commissars of the U.S.S.R. into the present V.I.E.M. A new building was erected in Leningrad; the staff was increased more than five times its size and a number of new laboratories were created especially for experimental biology, physics and chemistry.

Two years later, in 1934, the government decided to transfer the Institute to Moscow, the building in Leningrad to be a branch of a much larger Institute. More than 100,000,000 rubles were expended in building the new Institute. It was the largest, the best equipped, and staffed by the most brilliant scientists in the U.S.S.R. Consequently, it is one of the greatest of all medical institutes in the world today.

The scope of the Institute is wide and all-embracing. To get some idea of the work done we shall list the departments and laboratories. There are (1) the department of physiology; (2) neurophysiology; (3) physiology and physiopathology of the sense organs; (4) physiology and physiopathology of hearing; (5) electrophysiology; (6) barthermophysiolology; (7) protein hydrolizers; (8) department of pharmacology; (9) general pathology; (10) morphology; (11) laboratory for experimental embryology; (12) histopathology of the central nervous system; (13) cystology; (14) the department of photobiology; (15) physiological optics; (16) physiological chemistry; (17) microbiology and immunology; (18) microbiochemistry; (19) filtrable viruses; (20) brucellosis and tularemia; (21) medical parasitology; (22) organic chemistry.

The largest branch of the Moscow Institute is in Leningrad which consists of nine departments in which significant research is being carried out. In addition, scattered throughout the country, are various biological stations. In Pavlovo village there is a biological laboratory in which evolutionary physiology is being studied, particularly genetics and the higher nervous activity of arthropods. Another biological station is in Sukhumi in which monkey physiology is being studied and in which monkeys are being used in the study of various medical problems.

From time to time scientific expeditions are sent out from the V.I.E.M. to study various diseases in different parts of the Soviet Union and to investigate high altitude physiology. On the Institute's fiftieth anniversary a series of scientific sessions were organized and lectures were delivered by its members all over the country.

The principal problems under investigation in V.I.E.M. may be mentioned as follows:

1. Traumas, frostbite and burns. The problem of wound treatment is included as an essential part of the problem.

2. Infections and immunity. Most attention is paid to intestinal infections, then to virus diseases, especially those of the nervous system. Among children's diseases, diphtheria, scarlet fever, whooping cough and measles receive particular attention. Brucellosis and tularemia are also receiving attention.

3. The physiology of low atmospheric pressures. The effect of oxygen lack on protein metabolism, anoxemia and digestion, and changes in the nervous system under low barometric pressure are being studied.

4. Experimental studies on the causes of tuberculosis.

5. The causes of cancer.

6. The physiology and pathology of the heart and blood vessels.

7. Digestion.

8. Physiology and pathology of the higher nervous activity and the sense organs.

9. The role of the nervous system in various diseases.

10. The metabolism and chemistry of organic substances.

11. The biological function of physical factors such as ultra-high-frequency rays, and ultra-violet rays.

12. Physiochemistry of cells and tissues.

13. Evolutionary morphology.

All these problems are investigated jointly in the various laboratories, each specialist contributing from his own vast fund of knowledge and experience. Cooperative research or collective research is more productive and less time consuming.

Some of the significant discoveries to come out of the Maxim Gorki All-Union Institute of Experimental Medicine are:

1. Dr. N. N. Anichkov's work on arteriosclerosis. In his experiments Anichkov disclosed the mechanism whereby lime deposits are formed on the arch of the aorta.

2. Dr. B. Laventiev demonstrated the detailed structure of the vegetative nervous system and conducted a series of minute investigations on the nervous tissue connected with blood vessels, as well as on the connections between the carotid sinus and the blood vessels associated with it.

3. Drs. A. E. Braunstein and I. Kritsman have discovered new processes by which amino acids are formed.

4. Dr. A. G. Gurewitsch discovered mitogenetic radiation and demonstrated that it varied in intensity in the biological activity of the various organs and tissues including the blood.

5. Dr. Alexei D. Speransky showed the intimate part the nervous system plays in various infectious diseases, and devised methods of treatment to influence the nervous system in this respect to cure and alleviate these diseases.

6. Dr. A. V. Vishnevsky originated a number of successful methods for the treatment of wounds of the arms, legs, joints, the chest and the abdomen. He is particularly well known for devising the method of using novocaine as an anti-inflammatory agent, and as a powerful prophylactic agent against

traumatic shock. He also invented an ointment bandage which acts as an antiseptic and pain-allaying agent and prevents the dressing from adhering to the surface of the wound.

7. Dr. A. A. Zavarzin studied the evolution of the nervous system in the light of Darwin's theory of evolution.

8. Drs. E. N. Pavlosky, A. A. Smorodintsev, P. A. Petrishcheva, E. N. Levkovich and M. P. Chumakov studied the parasitology, diagnosis, treatment and prevention of seasonal neuro-virus encephalitis.

During the Second World War, V.I.E.M. contributed much to the war effort by investigating medical and surgical problems connected with warfare. The clinic of nervous diseases concerned itself with practical investigations in neurosurgery, particularly in discovering the methods of using sulfa drugs in the treatment of infections of the brain and nervous system, studying dangerous complications of skull and brain wounds, and the use of blood-clotting agents such as thrombin in brain surgery.

Dr. Z. V. Yermolieva did important work in the prophylaxis of cholera. She also worked out methods for the production of penicillin and checking its efficacy in the treatment of wound infections and wound sepsis. She also worked out new methods for the production of gramacidin and its use in various wound infections.

Drs. Drobyshevskaya and Smorodintsev worked out methods of rapid diagnosis of typhus and thus helped to check its spread. Dr. Chumakov perfected a more rapid method of diagnosing virus infections of the nervous system. A group of biophysicists under Dr. G. M. Frank studied the use of specially designed ultra-violet ray lamps for bacteria-killing action. These lamps were successfully used in various evacuation hospitals and assisted greatly in reducing the incidence of infection.

After the war the Institute returned to its research problems with renewed vigor. Of the principal scientific and practical problems which are at present receiving attention may be mentioned the following:

Dr. L. M. Khatenever and his associates have formulated methods of rapid diagnosis of tularemia. He has also produced an anti-tularemia vaccine which has thus far given very good results.

Dr. Gurewitch is continuing his work of mitogenetic radiation and is applying his discoveries to new fields, particularly the early diagnosis of wound infection. The physiology of higher nervous activity is receiving attention at the hands of the pupils of the late Dr. Pavlov. Dr. Shabad is doing some significant experimental work on the causes of cancer.

Work is now under way to increase the research facilities of V.I.E.M. The Council of People's Commissars of the U.S.S.R. have decided to establish an Academy of Medicine. The present All-Union Institute of Experimental Medicine will be divided into a number of independent research institutes which will go to form the Academy of Medicine.

The Academy will eventually comprise twenty-five research institutes. There will be three departments: the department of medico-biologic sciences, the department of clinical medicine, and the department of microbiology, epidemiology and hygiene. There will be many smaller departments which will go into making up the three main departments. Already plans are under way to undertake research along a score of different fronts of medical and biological knowledge. The greatest medical and scientific minds in the Soviet Union are joining in this new work, and there is no doubt that much of great value will come from this new research organization.

Part Three

A GALLERY OF RUSSIAN DOCTORS

XXXIV

NIKOLAI F. GAMALEYA

THE greatest microbe hunter in the Soviet Union is Nikolai Fedorvich Gamaleya, pupil and later colleague of the Father of Bacteriology, Louis Pasteur. Today Dr. Gamaleya is the Father of Bacteriology in Russia and its leading pioneer in the fight on microbial diseases. Now more than eighty-six years old he has taken his place with the all-time great in Russian medicine. It was he who in 1886 organized in Odessa the world's first inoculation center against rabies; he pioneered in his native land in establishing measures of prophylaxis and control against all the common infectious diseases.

N. F. Gamaleya was born in Odessa in 1859 and at an early age manifested interest in the natural sciences and medicine. In 1880 he was graduated from the University of Odessa, majoring in the natural sciences. Four years later he received his degree in medicine from the Military Medical Academy of St. Petersburg and entered medical practice in which he was successful from the start.

However, it was research which eventually engaged his attention, becoming interested in the new science of bacteriology. In 1881 Pasteur had announced his method of inoculating against rabies and in 1885 applied it successfully for the first time. Among those in Russia to become interested in this new method was Gamaleya and in 1886 the Odessa Medical Society sent him to the Pasteur Institute to study Pasteur's method. In a short time Dr. Gamaleya mastered the Pasteur technique and returned to Russia to put it into opera-

221

tion. He established a center for the treatment of rabies, to which other Russian physicians came to learn his method. Within a few years other rabies centers were established throughout Russia.

Although the study of rabies was Gamaleya's first interest, other infectious diseases soon claimed his interest and attention. He was the first Russian physician to devote himself to epidemiology and to the development of practical measures. The three most widespread infectious diseases at that time were plague, cholera and smallpox, and these claimed his immediate attention. He instituted measures of prophlyaxis and control. He was successful in fighting the plague and cholera in Transcaucasia and southern Russia, and by controlling the water supply accomplished a great deal in decreasing the incidence of these diseases. His book *Cholera and How to Combat It* became a classic in its field and taught other physicians practical bacteriological and sanitary measures in preventing the spread of this disease and bringing it under control.

The terror of the plague also claimed his attention. He initiated a campaign for the extermination of rats, the known carriers of this disease. In 1902 to 1904 he started practical methods of eliminating the plague in Odessa and southern Russia by a thorough extermination of the rats in the port of Odessa, the first time in Russian history that this was accomplished. At the same time he turned his attention to the louse, the carrier of typhus. He stressed the importance of delousing to prevent the spread of this dread disease.

The third great interest in Gamaleya's life was smallpox which at that time was killing and scarring hundreds of thousands of Russians. From 1910 to 1929 he was in charge of the Jenner Institute in Leningrad where he perfected and introduced methods of preparing smallpox vaccine and spreading its use throughout the country. In 1917 he was instrumental in making vaccination against smallpox com-

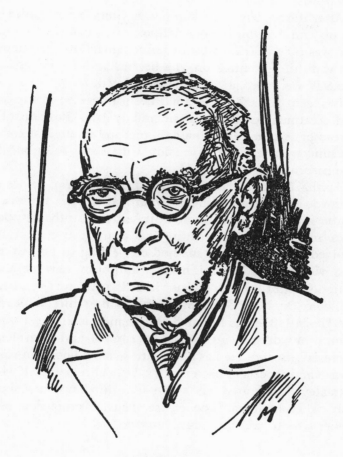

N. F. GAMALEYA

pulsory in Russia through his book *Vaccination Against Smallpox.*

After the Soviets came into power Gamaleya organized the supply and distribution of smallpox vaccine to the Red Army and was thus instrumental in reducing the disease almost to the vanishing point. From the beginning his services to the U.S.S.R. were recognized and appreciated.

In recent years Gamaleya has been interested in the causes and treatment of tuberculosis and grippe. To control the spread of grippe he originated a method in 1933 of treating the mucous membrane of the nose with a soap solution which was used with great success.

At the beginning of the Second World War he went to Borovoe in western Siberia where a famous tuberculosis center is situated. He devoted himself to a study of tuberculosis and methods of treating this disease, and in time he evolved his own specific method of treating it. From reports in Soviet medical journals his first tests of his new method on patients with tuberculosis has yielded satisfactory results.

Today Dr. N. F. Gamaleya is the leading microbiologist in the U.S.S.R. He has founded and headed many scientific organizations devoted to the study, control and treatment of bacterial diseases. He has also written many books on various phases and aspects of bacteriology. On February 18, 1944, Dr. Gamaleya celebrated his eighty-fifth birthday and sixtieth year as a physician. The entire medical profession of the Soviet Union paid him great homage.

XXXV

NIKOLAI NILOVICH BURDENKO

THE leading brain surgeon in the Soviet Union was also the Chief Surgeon of the Red Army. Nikolai Nilovich Burdenko at the age of sixty-five went out into the field with the army to do his part in helping to win the war. He worked under the severest conditions, in extreme cold, without light and water, to perform some of the most brilliant brain and nerve surgery in the late war.

Dr. Burdenko was used to war. He had been in two other wars: the Russo-Japanese War of 1904 in which, while still a medical student, he volunteered and served with great distinction as a medical assistant in the field. In the First World War he served as consulting surgeon of the Red Cross, and in 1917 he was appointed chief of the ambulance service of the Russian army.

In the Russo-Japanese War he received the Cross of St. George for bravery in action. Following his demobilization he completed his medical studies at Yuriev Derpt University. From 1906 to 1912 he rose from house surgeon to assistant professor of surgery at this university. In 1912 he was made full professor. Rapidly he established a reputation for himself as a brilliant brain and nerve surgeon, the best in Russia.

Following the First World War Burdenko refused offers of positions with the leading universities in order to devote himself to the study of shock in which he had become very much interested. He did much to further the understanding of this vexing problem in surgery and as a result of his discoveries a great many lives were saved which otherwise would have been lost.

Following his work with shock he received an appointment at the medical school of the University of Voronezh which he held for three years and where he did some of his most significant research in nerve and brain surgery.

He then returned to Moscow for a second time where medical opportunities were greater for neurosurgical work. In Moscow he laid the foundations of Russian neurosurgery. He became the greatest brain surgeon in the U.S.S.R. and one of the greatest in the world. For his accomplishments in this difficult field he was awarded the highest title of honor in the Soviet Union, Hero of Socialist Labor, which carries with it the Order of Lenin. He became a deputy to the Supreme Soviet of the U.S.S.R. and president of the Scientific Medical Council of the People's Commissariat of Public Health.

Burdenko was also a great clinical teacher. One of his most brilliant students is Vladimir V. Lebedenko who has rapidly assumed a place as a great neurosurgeon and whose fame has spread to other countries.

He was a modest man, giving credit to his associates and students. When he was awarded the Hero of Socialist Labor, he wrote: "My reward is the reward of all Soviet surgery. Soviet surgeons are working as one united front, both in the fighting areas and deep in the rear of the country. One is proud to be a member of such a brilliant collective and to occupy, because of historical conditions, one of its most responsible posts. This is how I regard the title of Hero of Socialist Labor bestowed on me by the Soviet government."

Burdenko was always an indefatigable worker. He remained with a problem in the operating room, in the clinic and in the laboratory until it was concluded. He often came down to work three o'clock in the morning. He had no regular hours. He worked at all hours because he had so much work to do.

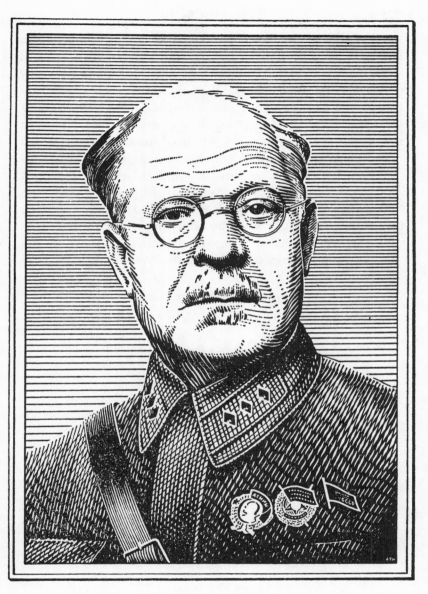

Nikolai N. Burdenko

Nikolai N. Burdenko has received recognition and honors from all parts of the world. He was a member of various foreign surgical associations, among them the Paris Academy of Surgery, the British Royal Society of Medicine and the International College of Surgeons. He bore these honors gracefully and modestly. Regarding these honors he said, "This, in my person, is an honor to the whole of Russian science which in the general opinion of British medical circles and American scientists occupies a foremost and in several respects a leading position. I have always endeavored to bring high aims, energy, and a spirit of restless endeavor to my work, and to inspire my colleagues with the same ideals. This spirit arose from the necessity of working intensely and selflessly for my country, both in times of peace and in the perilous war days."

XXXVI

SERGEI S. YUDIN

IN Moscow, on March 23, 1930, a young engineer tried to kill himself by cutting the arteries of his elbows. He was rushed to the Skilfassovsky Institute, Moscow's largest first-aid station, and brought in nearly dead from shock and loss of blood. An ordinary serum injection failed and no blood donor was available. Dr. Sergei S. Yudin then made an unprecedented transfusion. Six hours before, an old man had been brought in dead with a fractured skull. His blood was removed and nearly three-quarters of a pint suitably treated, was injected into the young man's veins. Two days later the would-be suicide left the hospital cured and well. He was the first of hundreds of men alive today because of Dr. Yudin's work.

In time Dr. Yudin learned many interesting things about human blood. He found, for instance, that in sudden, painless death the blood stays liquid in the human veins and will flow out by gravity even twenty-four hours after death. A lingering and painful death has a tendency to thicken the blood and form blood clots, rendering it unfit for transfusion purposes.

The Soviet government has sanctioned Dr. Yudin's work and it has been thoroughly systematized. All cases of sudden death which occur among the 3,000,000 population of the Russian capital are rushed to the Skilfassovsky Emergency Hospital, where the blood is collected, and if no immediate use for it is found it is stored for future use after sodium citrate has been added. The blood is kept in refrigerators.

Sergei S. Yudin, one of the greatest of Soviet surgeons, was born in 1892, and at the age of twenty-two was graduated from the medical school of Moscow University. His graduation came at a time when the First World War was getting under way and he went off to war as a medical officer in the Imperial Russian army. Following his discharge from the army, Yudin became a Zemstvo physician and was assigned to the Zakharino sanatorium, a short distance from Moscow. He had always been interested in surgery and at the sanatorium performed his first operations. In 1922 he was transferred to Serpukhovski, where in the hospital of that city he continued his surgical work, particularly in surgery of the stomach, with great success and distinction. Young Dr. Yudin regularly presented case reports before the Moscow Surgical Society and his reputation as a gastric surgeon soon spread. He attracted many other surgeons from various parts of Russia who came to learn his methods of treating perforated and bleeding ulcers.

For four years Dr. Yudin continued his remarkable work at Serpukhovski, at the end of which time the government sent him abroad to study surgical methods in the United States. In 1926 Dr. Yudin made a tour of American hospitals and became acquainted with the leading American surgeons, among them, the Mayos, Crile, Kelly, Cushing and Babcock. This trip resulted in a book, *A Guest of American Surgeons*, which did much to acquaint Russian surgeons with the work that American surgeons were doing.

In 1928 Dr. Yudin became the director of surgery of the Skilfassovsky Institute for Traumatic Diseases, a 700-bed hospital in Moscow, with a medical staff of 200 surgeons, to which all emergency cases are brought. This hospital is one of the most remarkable in the world, and all other great cities might do well to establish emergency hospitals patterned after it. It has thirteen ambulances on twenty-four-hour duty and four substations in various parts of the city. About 60,-

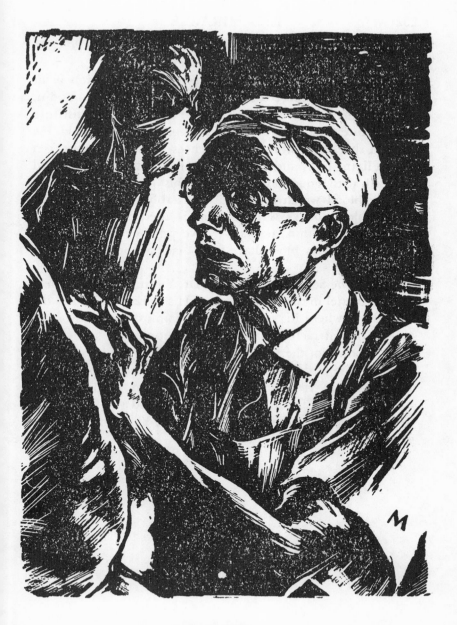

SERGEI S. YUDIN

000 cases of an emergency nature are treated here a year. For a surgeon the work is of the greatest value.

In all traumatic or accident cases blood transfusion is an essential part of the treatment. For this reason Dr. Yudin, early during his directorship of the Skilfassovsky Institute became interested in the biochemical properties of blood. He learned that there were no differences between blood taken from a living body and that taken from a cadaver. Both could be used with good results. It was his pioneer work with cadaver blood which did much to establish the widespread use of blood banks. His method is used throughout the U.S.S.R. and within the past twelve years over 5,000 transfusions of cadaver blood have been made at the Skilfassovsky Institute.

During the Second World War Dr. Yudin served as a lieutenant colonel in the medical corps. His work took him to the front lines where his treatment of complex fractures of the extremities attracted favorable attention. The army conferred upon him the Order of the Red Star, the government gave him the Order of Stalin. His work has been appreciated abroad, for in 1943 he was given honorary fellowships in both the American College of Surgeons and the Royal College of Surgeons of England. Dr. Sergei S. Yudin is one of the greatest surgeons of all time.

XXXVII

LINA SOLOMONOVA STERN

THE leading woman physician in the Soviet Union is Lina Solomonova Stern. She received her medical education in Switzerland and during her medical student days she became very much interested in physiology. In 1903 she received her doctor of medicine degree, her thesis being a physiological study of uterine contractions. One year later she entered the Department of Physiology of the University of Geneva as assistant to Professor Prevost. Within two years she rose to the rank of lecturer. While carrying on her teaching duties she did considerable research in physiology, publishing papers on the results of her investigations.

In 1917 she turned her attentions to physiological chemistry and became the first professor in that science in the University of Geneva. Her work was mainly concerned with the biochemistry and physiology of the central nervous system. She performed many experiments on cerebral irritants, also on the effects of various drugs such as curare on the cerebellum.

Although a Russian, she had spent quite a few years in Geneva. When the Soviets came into power they recognized her scientific achievements. In 1925 she was invited to come to the Second Moscow University as Professor of Physiology. She had a rather difficult time adjusting to her new surroundings. She met with antagonism among her colleagues because of her reputation and because she had been away from home for so many years, but she managed to overcome these obstacles and resume her studies and researches in a most fruitful manner.

The scientific world of the Soviet Union was not without appreciation for her work. Within nine years after her acceptance of the chair of physiology a volume of more than 700 pages was published in her honor bearing the title, *Problems of Biology and Medicine,* which contained articles written by eminent scientists from every country in the world.

Dr. Stern has connections with many scientific institutions in which she does special research dealing with physiological problems. She is the head of the Scientific Research Institute of Physiology; she is in charge of the Department of General Physiology of the All-Union Institute of Experimental Medicine as well as of the Department of the Physiology of Growth of the Institute of the Protection of Motherhood and Infancy. In addition she carries on a rather full teaching program and is editor of the *Bulletin of Experimental Biology and Medicine.* She never has an idle moment. Every minute of her day is usefully occupied.

During the late war Dr. Stern, though a woman no longer young, devoted all her time and energies to war problems. She worked out practical applications of physiological principles to war medicine and surgery. She evolved a method for the treatment of shock, based on the principle of direct action on the nerve centers in cases where, because of certain barriers, the substance injected into the blood stream did not penetrate into the spinal fluid.

Another valuable contribution she made during the war was the following: It is well known that in shock the leading role is played by the autonomic nervous system and particularly by the sympathetic centers. Dr. Stern developed a method of stimulating these nerve centers by injecting a solution of potassium phosphate directly into the brain. She obtained excellent results and this method was widely adopted. She also developed a new method of treating tetanus or

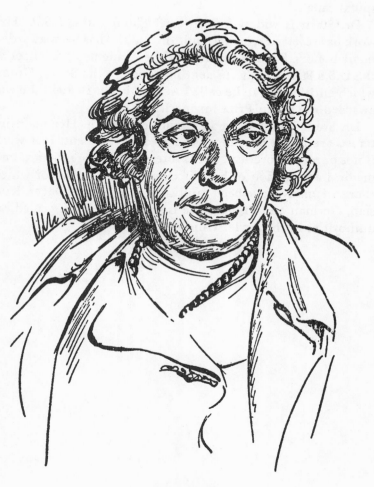

LINA S. STERN

lock-jaw by injecting anti-tetanus serum directly into the spinal canal.

Dr. Stern is widely known throughout the U.S.S.R. Her work has received wide recognition and she has been awarded many honors. She is a member of the Academy of Sciences of the U.S.S.R, the highest scientific honor in the Soviet Union which entitled her to be called Academician. In 1943 she was awarded the Stalin Prize for merit.

Dr. Stern is still active in scientific research. Her main interests are in the physiology of nervous treatment. Her work is not purely theoretical. She is interested in the practical and medical application of her discoveries. Her works, of which there are many, have been published in three languages, Russian, German and French. She is one of the leading medical authorities in the Soviet Union today.

XXXVIII

NIKOLAI NIKOLAEVICH PRIOROV

THE greatest expert on trauma, wounds and splintered bones in the Soviet Union is Nikolai Nikolaevich Priorov. He has done more to restore and rehabilitate the wounded and crippled in Russia than any other man. He is cunning with his hands in not only repairing crippled human beings, but also in fashioning and inventing prosthetics and devices to enable the severely injured to live and lead a normal life.

Priorov was born in Archangelsk in 1885. His early youth was spent in the north where he received his academic education and later his medical education at Tomsk, Siberia. Following his graduation he entered the Botkin Hospital in Moscow where he served as an assistant surgeon for two years. At the outbreak of the First World War he entered the army as a military surgeon. He served in this capacity from 1914 to 1919, transferring to the Red Army when that was organized.

He served with great distinction, attracting favorable attention because of his remarkable work in orthopedic and reconstructive surgery. As a reward for his services he was appointed Director of the Central Hospital for War Invalids. Here he further enhanced his reputation as an expert in trauma and injuries so that in 1921 he was appointed Director of the Central Institute of Traumatology and Orthopedic Surgery in Moscow, a position he still holds. During the years he has held this important position he has contributed much to the knowledge of wound and bone surgery. He has within recent years been elected President of the Society of Orthopedic, Traumatologic and Prosthetic Workers. This society is vitally concerned with evolving and making known the latest and most effective means of restoring and rehabilitating the wounded and crippled, not only as a result of the war, but also because of various accidents.

N. N. Priorov is a prolific and productive writer who has published well over a hundred papers on his specialties. His name is also widely associated with various devices to replace missing hands, arms, feet and legs. To mention but a few of these: he has invented a very ingenious device for persons who have lost the use of both hands and eyes, various apparatus and traction frames for the reduction and treatment of the most severe dislocations and fractures and a corset for the alleviation of severe spinal curvatures.

In addition to his various other duties Dr. Priorov is in charge of a hospital of 300 beds devoted exclusively to the treatment of the most serious of bone disorders. He has done remarkable work in the correction of club foot and the plastic reconstruction of victims of advanced poliomyelitis.

Still another duty that Dr. Priorov performs is that of Professor of Orthopedic Surgery at the First Moscow Medical Institute and also at the Postgraduate Institute for physicians. He trained some forty aspirants and internes from his Institute before the war who rendered valuable service in the field.

During the Second World War Dr. Priorov spent a great deal of time at the various war fronts. He was Chief Surgeon of the Evacuation Hospitals and this took him over a great part of the U.S.S.R. He also served as instructor in special war surgery and trained hundreds of surgeons to care for the seriously crippled and wounded. Previously he had distinguished himself in the Mongolian and Russo-Finnish Wars.

Lately, he headed a group of distinguished Soviet surgeons in a visit to the United States to observe American methods in traumatology and orthopedic surgery. He made a favorable impression on American surgeons with his skill and knowledge as well as his receptivity for American ideas in his spe-

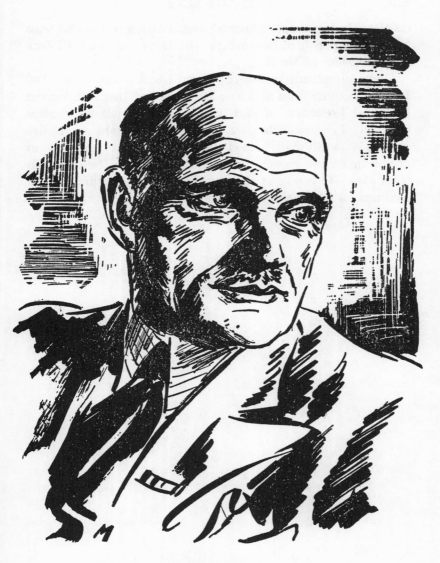

N. N. PRIOROV

cialties. He was amply honored by his own government who bestowed upon him two orders: the Order of the Red Star and the Order of Merit.

Upon his return to Moscow from his American visit Dr. Priorov became head of a new Hospital and Institute for the Care and Treatment of War Invalids in the outskirts of Moscow. Dr. Priorov feels that his most important work lies ahead. With his skill, knowledge and ingenuity there is no doubt that even greater accomplishments may be expected from him. He is one of the world's greatest Menders of the Maimed, of which the whole world needs many.

XXXIX

ANATOL ALEXANDROVICH SMORODINTSEV

O NE of the leading younger bacteriologists in Soviet medicine is Anatol Alexandrovich Smorodintsev. He invented a method of treating influenza with vaporized influenza anti-serum which has been widely adopted in the
United States. The inhalation of anti-serum has yielded extremely good results and it has been found of value not only
in curing influenza but also for preventing outbreaks of this
disease.

A. A. Smorodintsev was born in Birsk, a small town near
Ufa in the Bashkirian Republic, on September 19, 1901. His
father was a physician and young Anatol, after completing his
academic education in his home town, decided to become a
physician too. He received his medical degree in 1923 from
the University of Tomsk Medical School. The following year
he was called up for military service, after completing his in-
terneship at the Institute of Bacteriology in Tomsky. He
served as a specialist in bacteriology in the medical corps and
upon his demobilization went to Leningrad where he joined
the Pasteur Institute as a bacteriologist. By successive promo-
tions, he became head in 1933 of the Department of Bacteriology of the Institute. He was also connected with the
Institute of Experimental Medicine in which he carried out
researches in bacteriology which won him fame both in the
Soviet Union and abroad.

In 1934 a strange disease known as "toxic influenza" broke
out in the taiga country of the Far East. This ailment was
characterized by severe headaches, epileptoid seizures, high

temperature, dizziness, vomiting and coma. The mortality was high; and those who recovered were, for the most part, paralyzed.

In 1937 a group of physicians left for the taiga country to determine just what the disease was. They established the fact that it was spread by ticks. The following year Dr. Smorodintsev headed another group of investigators to study the so-called toxic influenza. He confirmed that it was spread by ticks but he also discovered several other interesting things about the disease. It appeared that the disease struck down only the road builders, the geologists and the lumberjacks whose work took them into the woods. More men were afflicted than women, particularly men past forty. Also, newcomers were more likely to become victims of this disease than the old-time inhabitants who seemed to have developed some sort of immunity to it through the years. Furthermore, the disease was not contagious, for those who came in contact with the victims did not fall ill.

Dr. Smorodintsev succeeded in establishing the fact that this so-called toxic influenza was a form of encephalitis and that it was transmitted by a filtrable virus. The virus affected the brain which brought on the symptoms of severe headaches, dizziness, fits and coma.

The next step was to develop means of combating this disease. Dr. Smorodintsev and his associates developed an anti-serum. The following year he led another group back to the taiga with an ample supply of vaccine to combat the disease. In one locality Dr. Smorodintsev and his associates vaccinated 925 men early in April before the disease made its appearance. As a control another group of 1,185 men were not vaccinated. Within the next three months they would know if the vaccine would work. And they did. In the vaccinated group only two very mild cases of the disease occurred. In the group which was not vaccinated there were twenty-seven severe cases of which seven died.

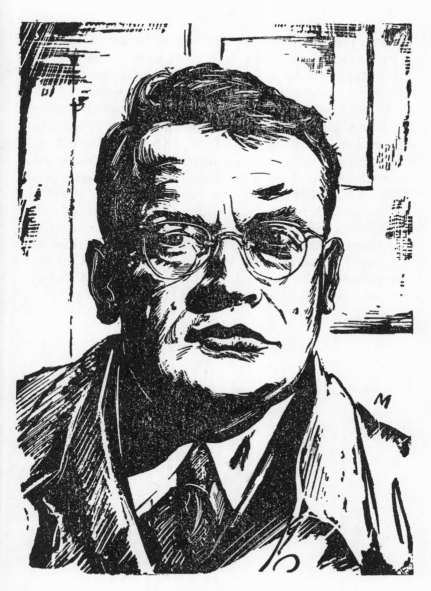

ANATOL A. SMORODINTSEV

The value of the vaccine was now established and it was widely used in that area. In a short time the disease was eradicated from the taiga and that country is now as safe as any in the Soviet Union in which to live and work.

Dr. Smorodintsev since then has been one of the busiest physicians in the U.S.S.R. Whenever there is an epidemic of any proportions in any part of the U.S.S.R. he is sent for to study it and devise measures to control it. He thus travels many thousands of miles every year. Recently he was a guest of the Rockefeller Institute for Medical Research where he discussed his methods of vaccination and immunization.

Although still a young man Dr. Smorodintsev is not without honors. He has received many prizes and awards for his researches in bacteriology. When the Stalin Award for Distinguished Service was established in 1941, Dr. A. A. Smorodintsev was the first to receive it.

XL

VALENTINE D. SOLOVIEV

O NE of the leading epidemiologists in the Soviet Union is
a young medical man, Dr. Valentine Dmitrievich Soloviev. He has done remarkable work in encephalitis, particularly that variety known as tick-borne encephalitis, for
which he helped devise a vaccine which has been widely used
with very good results.

Valentine D. Soloviev was born in Sverdlovsky on October
20, 1907. He was adopted by a physician, Dr. Dmitri Soloviev,
when he was abandoned by his own parents whom he has
happily forgotten. Until his death in 1917 Dr. Soloviev took
the best care of his young protégé and instilled in him a love
for medicine and a desire to serve humanity. Following the
death of his foster father young Valentine took to the road
and finally came to Perm, later renamed Molotov, where at
the age of fourteen he found employment. Here he worked
first as a common day laborer and later as an electrician,
finding time to study for the latter occupation because of
his constant urge to improve his lot in life. He continued to
work as an electrician and study a great variety of subjects.
This reading stood him in good stead for when he later applied for admission to the University of Perm, he was accepted at once in spite of the fact that his preliminary education was extremely sketchy. He enlisted in the liberal arts
course for he wanted a firm and sound educational basis upon
which to build his later scientific training. He graduated in
1932 and went at once to Moscow to study medicine. In 1936
he received his doctor's degree in medicine.

He completed his military service with distinction and in 1939 became research director of the Moscow Institute of Microbiology. During the late war he served as an epidemiologist with the Pacific fleet and in this capacity did a great deal of research in virus diseases and devised means of controlling them in the armed forces.

When he was demobilized, Dr. Soloviev returned to the Central Institute of Microbiology and Epidemiology as research director and in this position, which he has held since, he has done some of the most remarkable work in his specialty.

Under his direction at the Institute are produced all the vaccines and sera which are used by the armed forces and civilian populations of the Soviet Union. The division which Dr. Soloviev heads is made up of seven departments in which research in all phases of bacteriology and epidemiology are constantly being carried out. Investigations in immunity have brought many important procedures to light which are now widely used for the prevention of many contagious diseases.

Virus diseases have been the special province of Dr. Soloviev. It was this interest in viruses which brought about his meeting Antonina Konstantinovna Shubladze, a beautiful young virus expert whom he married and who now works at his laboratory with him.

The research division which Dr. Soloviev heads consists of twenty-two scientists, four aspirants and many laboratory assistants. Research is constantly being carried out on many subjects; papers are being published in the leading scientific and medical journals announcing the discovery of new facts and methods of treatment. Very significant researches have been carried out on intestinal diseases, influenza and children's diseases, all under the direction and supervision of young Dr. Soloviev.

The main interest of Dr. Soloviev is still encephalitis, in which he has done some very remarkable investigations.

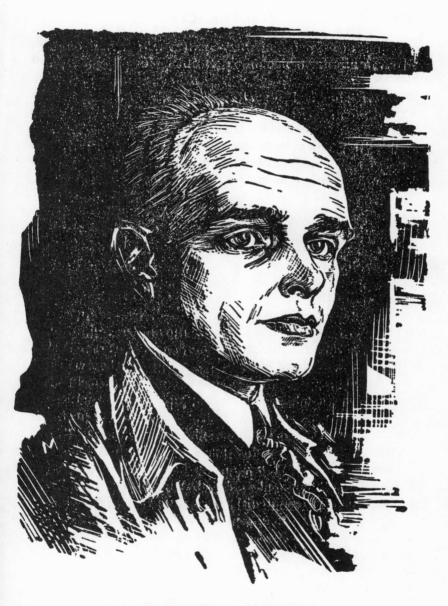

VALENTINE D. SOLOVIEV

Under his immediate supervision his staff has carried on experiments in demyelinated encephalitis, a very serious virus disease of the nervous system. Much of great value in diagnosis and pathology of this disease has already come to light.

For his scientific discoveries Dr. Soloviev was awarded in 1941 the Stalin Award for Distinguished Service. In 1942 he was given the degree of Doctor of Science and made a full Professor of Epidemiology. He continues to distinguish himself, his profession and his country.

XLI

EUGENE N. PAVLOVSKI

WHEN the Soviet Union realized the great importance that insects played in the transmission of disease it went about organizing ways and means to combat this menace. The Institute of Experimental Medicine was reorganized along modern lines and transferred to the All-Union Institute of Experimental Medicine in Moscow. One of the most important departments in this newly organized medical institution was that of medical parasitology, and the man chosen to head it was Dr. Eugene N. Pavlovski, the greatest parasitologist in the U.S.S.R.

Pavlovski was born in Biryuche, in the Gubernia of Voronezh, Russia, on February 22, 1884, the son of a school teacher. He had always been interested in the natural sciences and he knew even as a boy what he wanted most to do in life. He wanted to apply a practical knowledge of the natural sciences to medicine. For this reason he prepared himself for the Military Medical Academy at St. Petersburg where he desired particularly to study under Dr. N. A. Kholodovski, Russia's leading biologist at that time. Pavlovski was one of the most brilliant students in his preparatory school where he won a gold medal. He entered the medical school in 1903, where, as a student a year later, he attracted the notice of his idol, Dr. Kholodovski. The eminent biologist was much intrigued by the enthusiasm of the young medical student and he assigned him a most prosaic problem, the anatomy of the human louse. Pavlovski went about this task with great thoroughness and wrote two papers on the subject which attracted favorable attention.

Pavlovski demonstrated at an early age that his main object in life was the study of insect-borne disease, and the early interest in the louse soon spread to a study of other insects, enemies of man because they spread often fatal ailments. In 1908, while still a student at the medical school, he went on his first expedition to Samarkand to undertake a study of poisonous fish. This was the first of ninety such expeditions all over the world to study conditions which contribute to the disease producing elements of mankind. As a result of these expeditions much of great value in public health measures has been learned and put into execution.

In 1909 Pavlovski graduated from the academy, and within the next five years he received his doctor's degree in medicine, a master's degree in zoology and an appointment as assistant in zoology and comparative anatomy at his alma mater.

Dr. Pavlovski was not content to lead an ivory tower existence. The whole world was his province and he felt that much was to be gained in intercourse with other scientists. In 1914 he was successful in getting a traveling scholarship which took him all over Europe and Africa where he visited various biological and zoological institutions and stations. During this trip he met many famous physicians, particularly Dr. C. Nicolle at the Pasteur Institute in Tunis. This trip was most successful from a productive point of view. He became intensely interested in scorpions; he wrote a comprehensive monograph on the comparative anatomy of the scorpion which attracted favorable attention and which won him an award.

Before he could complete his European trip the First World War broke out and he returned to Russia where he served in the medical corps of the army with great distinction.

Following the Revolution Pavlovski played an important

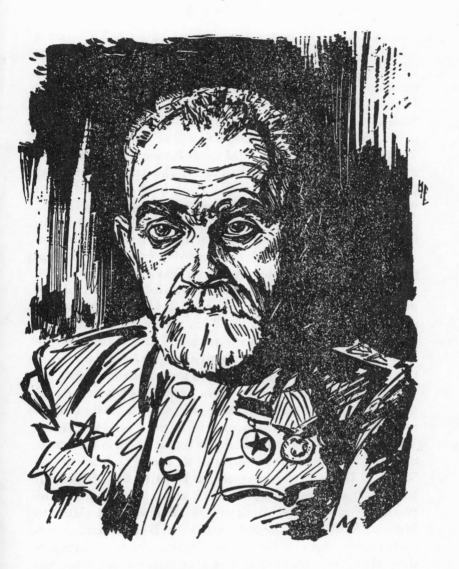

EUGENE N. PAVLOVSKI

role in helping to establish medicine in the U.S.S.R. on a sound and scientific basis. He was by now without a peer as the premier parasitologist in Russia. He helped to organize the Department of General Biology and Parasitology of the Military Medical Academy of the Red Army in Leningrad. This became the leading school for the training of medical parasitologists and entomologists in the Soviet Union. Pavlovski became the Father of Medical Parasitology in the new government and was responsible for the training of many competent medical parasitologists who have done marvelous work in curbing the spread of disease by insect pests. During the Second World War Pavlovski was influential in preventing the spread of disease among the troops. His contribution to helping the Russians win a great victory was felt and appreciated. Just one contribution of Pavlovski in this connection might be mentioned. He devised methods of impregnating clothing against insect bites, which helped to ward off the phlebotomus fly. This was of the greatest importance for Red Army units stationed and fighting in localities where this fly spread phlebotomus fever. Deaths from this ailment were reduced almost to the vanishing point.

Eugene N. Pavlovski is one of the greatest of Soviet medical men today. He is not without honor, for the Soviets adore men of scientific achievement. He is the president of the Tadzhik branch of the Academy of Sciences. He is an Academician, director of the Institute of Zoology, Academy of Sciences, U.S.S.R., director of the Department of General Biology and Parasitology, V.I.E.M. and director of the Department of General Biology and Parasitology, Military Medical Academy of the Red Army. He is the bearer of several orders and has honorary degrees from universities throughout the world. But first and foremost he is a great doctor.

Part Four

THE PROMISE OF THE FUTURE

XLII

SOCIALIZED MEDICINE

WHAT is socialized medicine? It is a form of medicine in which the state exerts control over physicians and all matters pertaining to medicine and its practice. Russia is the outstanding example of a country in which socialized medicine is practiced today. Russia, with a population of approximately 170,000,000 people, now has 150,000 doctors as compared with our 120,000 physicians for 130,000,000 people. In addition, Russia has 300,000 trained medical aids known as *feldshars,* as well as midwives and nurses. Some 800,000 hospital beds are available in Russia; in the United States in 1941 there were 1,324,381.

The sixty medical schools in the Soviet Union are comparable with our seventy-seven Grade-A schools in quality. Medical school tuition in Russia is free and all living needs are provided the students who, after graduation, are sent to rural communities to practice for three years. At the end of that period they are free to select a location for carrying on their profession, but there is no private practice as it is understood in the United States. All physicians are employees of the state. They are free, however, to specialize if they choose, or devote themselves to research in connection with, or independent of, their regular work.

The effectiveness of the U.S.S.R.'s system of training medical men is evidenced by the great contributions that Soviet physicians and surgeons have made to medicine within the past few decades. Some of the most remarkable accomplish-

255

ments in medicine have taken place in Russia, and these have received world-wide recognition.

In the Soviet Union a physician's average yearly salary is between $1,500 and $3,500, which is more than an adequate income in Russia. In addition, each doctor receives an annual four week's vacation with pay, three month's postgraduate work at government expense every three years, and, like all other Soviet citizens, is eligible for sick benefits and old age pensions.

While there is no other country like Russia in which medicine is so thoroughly under state control, tendencies toward the socialization of medicine are becoming manifested in other countries throughout the world. In Belgium a struggle is in progress between the government and the medical profession. In effect, the proposed law of social insurance involves the loss of almost all free practice. At present, there are in Belgium 2,600,000 persons under social insurance. If the draft of the law is adopted it will mean that 96.5 per cent of the population will be under social insurance, and this will lead to state medicine such as exists in Russia. France is undergoing a similar experience.

In Brazil the President recently signed two decrees which tend toward the socialization of medicine in that country. The first decree establishes the minimum sum to be paid to a doctor for professional services rendered by them as employees in private medical organizations. The professional services are distributed in many specialties. The same decree states the minimum duration of work which varies from four to eight hours a day, with a weekly maximum of twenty-four hours and a scale which introduces a basis for variation important to cities and states. The decree specifies that, in cases of disagreement between a private patient and the physician about the sum to be collected for medical care, when the case goes to court and the sum claimed is not more than $500, the amount demanded should be considered a definite right of the physician in accordance with the record on his books. To enjoy this right the physician is obliged to have routine record books with full informative entries in order to make possible the necessary investigations by the judge. This decree for the practice of medicine corresponds to the minimum wage and salary law in labor legislation. In many known cases the federal government and the state and municipal administrations pay their medical employees salaries that are substantially inferior to the minimum established by the new decree.

The second decree is of more sweeping power. This decree institutes councils of medicine "to maintain the exact observance of the principles of professional ethics in the practice of medicine." This provides for a federal council in the capital of the country and a regional council in every state or federal territory. The regional councils are composed of five members elected for three years by the secret vote of the physicians regularly registered in the state or territory. The federal council consists of seven members elected by secret vote for a five-year period. The principal functions of the councils are:

1. To maintain a register of the physicians legally entitled to practice medicine in the state or territory.

2. To judge the cases of infringement of the principles of medical ethics and impose the necessary penalties.

3. To exercise the right of arbitration in cases in which physicians are involved professionally.

In the United States legislation has been proposed in the Senate and House of Representatives which would also attempt to socialize medical practice. The Wagner-Murray-Dingell Bill has aroused a great deal of debate pro and con. This bill provides:

1. Grants-in-aid to states for the treatment and control of venereal disease and tuberculosis and the extension of the Public Health Service.

2. An extension of maternal and child health services through grants-in-aid to states.

3. Grants-in-aid to states to provide medical care for the needy.

4. Health services for all Social Security beneficiaries and all of their dependents.

5. Federal funds to subsidize medical research and education.

SECTION BY SECTION ANALYSIS
of
Senate Bill 1050—H. R. Bill 3293

SECTION I.—GRANTS AND LOANS FOR STUDIES OF HEALTH FACILITIES AND FOR HOSPITAL CONSTRUCTION.

Part 1. Provides for Surveys and Planning.

A. Purposes are to grant to states up to 50 per cent of cost of approved plans for surveys which will
   1. Result in evaluation of present hospital facilities.
   2. Canvass needs for new construction.
   3. Result in the development of programs for hospital projects.

B. Appropriates $5,000,000 to be expended by June 30, 1055.

C. Financed by appropriations from general revenues.

D. Authority: Surgeon-General of the Public Health Service.

Part 2. Hospital and Medical Facilities Construction.

A. Authorizes grants or loans to states, other governmental agencies and to non-profit organizations of
   1. From 25 per cent—50 per cent of project costs.
   2. Additional federal loans of 25 per cent of project costs.

B. Appropriations for construction:
  1. Fiscal year ending June 30, 1946—$50,000,000.
  2. For succeeding 9 fiscal years—$900,000,000.
C. Appropriations for state administration:
  1. Additional for administrative grants to states for fiscal year ending June 30, 1945—$5,000,000.
  2. Sufficient sums for the 9 succeeding fiscal years.
D. Appropriation for federal administration:
  1. Additional for administration by Surgeon General —$2,000,000.
E. Source of funds—general revenues.
F. Administration: Supervised by U. S. Surgeon General.

SECTION II.—GRANTS TO STATES FOR PUBLIC HEALTH SERVICES.
A. Purpose is to extend public health services (specifically to provide for control of venereal disease and tuberculosis and including also customary and accepted functions of public health services).
B. Appropriations for:
  1. Venereal diseases: not specified.
  2. Tuberculosis control:
    a. For fiscal year ending June 30, 1945—$10,000,000;
    b. For each fiscal year thereafter, sufficient sums.
  3. Improving public health services, especially in economically depressed areas and communities, training of personnel for state and local public health work, etc.
    a. For each fiscal year, beginning with fiscal year ending June 30, 1946 sufficient sums.
      1. Of the sum appropriated for each fiscal year an amount not to exceed $5,000,000 shall be available to the Surgeon General for demonstrations, training of personnel, cost of pay.

allowances, traveling expenses of commissioned officers and other personnel assisting
the states in carrying out the program.
C. Source of funds—from general revenues.
  a. Grants may amount to from 25 to 75 percent of
  amounts expended by states.
D. Authority—supervision of Surgeon General of the
Public Health Service.

SECTION III.—GRANTS TO STATES FOR MATERNAL
AND CHILD HEALTH AND WELFARE SERVICES.
A. Maternal and child health services.
  1. Extends services and facilities for promoting the
  health of mothers and children.
B. Services for crippled children.
  1. To extend and improve medical, surgical corrective
  services, hospital and after care for crippled and
  physically handicapped children.
C. Appropriations: For each fiscal year (beginning with
  fiscal year ending June 30, 1946) sufficient sums to
  carry out the purposes.
D. Child Welfare services.
  1. To extend and strengthen existing child welfare
  services needed for the prevention and control of
  child dependency, neglect, delinquency and to
  suitable care and protection for children with
  parental care.
E. Appropriations.
  1. For each of the fiscal years ending June 30, 1946 and
  June 30, 1947—$15,000,000.
  2. Sufficient sums for each fiscal year thereafter.
  3. For administrative expenses: For each fiscal year (beginning with the fiscal year ending June 30, 1946)
  sufficient sums.

F. Source of funds—general revenues.
   1. Grants may amount to from 25 to 75 per cent of the amounts expended.
G. Administration: Chief of Children's Bureau of the Department of Labor.

SECTION IV.—COMPREHENSIVE PUBLIC ASSIST-
ANCE PROGRAM (GRANTS TO STATES AFTER
JUNE 30, 1945).
   A. Financial assistance for needy, aged, blind, dependent children under 18 years of age. May also include medical care for needy individuals and payments for the care of needy children in foster homes.
   B. Appropriations: sufficient sums for each fiscal year (beginning with the fiscal year ending June 30, 1946).
   C. Source of funds—general revenues.
      1. Grants may amount to from 50 to 75 per cent of amounts expended.
   D. Administration—States: Subject to approval by Social Security Board.

SECTION V.—A NATIONAL SYSTEM OF EMPLOY-
MENT OFFICES.
   Provides for creation of United States Employment Service, on the Social Security Board. Six months after termination of war present U. S. Employment Service and all related activities of War Manpower Commission are to be transferred to new Employment Service.
   Function of the proposed service will be to establish Federal Employment offices all over the United States, manned by federal personnel, to carry on the general reference, placement and informational work of such offices.

SECTION VI.—NATIONAL SOCIAL INSURANCE SYS-
TEM.

Part 1. Prepared Medical Care Insurance.
  A. Medical and Hospital Care
    1. Benefits include services of physicians, specialists, dentists, and nurses; use of laboratory and x-ray equipment: and hospitalization.
    2. Duration of hospitalization benefits: 60 days maximum per year (possibly 120 days if resources of insurance fund are sufficient).
    3. Coverage: Employees and dependents, and self-employed.
  B. Grants-in-aid for medical education, research and prevention of disease and disability, including rehabilitation of veterans and disabled persons.
  C. Administration: U. S. Surgeon General (under supervision of Federal Security Administrator).

Within the National Social Insurance Trust Fund, there is created a Personal Health Services Account. Into this account is to be paid 3 per cent of all wages and earnings taxed under this Act. It is estimated that this will provide $3,142,-000,000 annually to help pay for these services.

Part 2. Unemployment and Temporary Disability Insurance.
  A. Unemployment benefits:
    1. Up to $30 per week.
    2. Waiting periods: 1 week.
    3. Duration: 26 weeks and possibly 52 weeks.
    4. Coverage: Employees, except self-employed.
  B. Temporary Disability Benefits:
    1. Up to $30 per week.
    2. Waiting period: 1 week.
    3. Duration: 26 weeks.
    4. Coverage: Employees and dependents, except self-employed.
  C. Administration: Social Security Board.

Part 3. Retirement, Survivors and Extended (Permanent) Disability Insurance Benefits.

A. Persons covered would be those now covered under Old-Age and Survivors' insurance system, and—agricultural workers, domestic workers, seamen, employees of non-profit institutions, professional persons, small business men and farmers.

B. Increase of Old Age Social Insurance benefits:
1. Benefit formula changed to provide for general increases.
2. Maximum: Increased from $85 to $120 per month.
3. Minimum: Increased from $10 to $20 per month.
   a. $30 if insured has dependent wife over 60.

Note: 1. Eligibility age for women reduced from 65 to 60 years.
2. Permits earnings up to $25 per month in addition to benefits.

C. Extended (permanent) disability benefits (where insured worker is totally disabled for 6 months before reaching retirement age).
1. Benefit scale same as under Old Age Social Insurance.
2. If the service of an attendant is necessary by reason of disability, a maximum of $25 a month may be granted in addition.

D. Lump sum death benefit payments:
1. Payments equal to 6 times the primary old-age benefit of deceased worker:
(a) To spouse, or (b) other person to the extent of expense incurred in meeting burial cost of the deceased.

E. Parents' Insurance Benefits.
1. Monthly payments equal one-half of primary benefit of deceased person: (a) Male at 65, (b) Female at 60.

F. Administration: Social Security Board.

SECTION VII.—NATIONAL SOCIAL INSURANCE TRUST FUND

A. Created to receive all existing assets credited to the Federal Old Age and Survivors' Insurance system.

B. May receive Unemployment Compensation reserves of the several states where transfer is approved by a state legislature. The bill also provides that: "In return for the assumption by the Federal Government of the obligation to pay unemployment benefits, a state shall be required, as a condition for the receipt of any grant or payment authorized under this Act . . . , to transfer to the National Social Insurance Trust Fund the unexpended balances in its unemployment fund. . . ."

C. Administration is by a Board of Trustees—Secretary of the Treasury, who will be the Managing Trustee, Secretary of Labor, and Chairman of the Social Security Board—which is directed to:

1. Hold the fund.

2. Establish separate accounts, as may be necessary.

3. Report to each regular session of Congress, or oftener if the Trustees are "of the opinion that during the ensuing five fiscal years the Trust Fund (or any separate account) will be excessively or unduly small."

4. To invest the fund as a single fund, "only in interest-bearing obligations of the United States" or guaranteed by it.

5. Pay, from time to time, into the Treasury, the amounts estimated to be needed during a three-month period for administrative expenses.

SECTION VIII.—CREDIT FOR MILITARY SERVICES.

A. Servicemen to be credited on the basis of $160 a month pay for each month of military service after September 7, 1939.

SECTION IX.—SOCIAL INSURANCE CONTRIBU-
TIONS.
  A. Taxes are based on earnings up to $3600 a year, begin-
  ning January 1, 1946.
    1. Employers are to contribute 4%.
    2. Employees are to contribute 4%.
    3. Self-employed are to contribute 5%.

NOTE: Self-employed are not covered for Unemployment
Compensation and Temporary Disability benefits, and therefore their contributions are less than the total of employer
and employee contributions.

The key provisions of the Wagner-Murray-Dingell Bill are
more comprehensive than any measures enacted into law in
any country thus far with the possible exception of the
U.S.S.R. Control over medical practice would be as complete
as it is in the Soviet Union. This bill would establish the
Surgeon General of the Public Health Service—under the direction of the Administrator of the Social Security Board,
would have full authority to:

  1. Hire doctors, specialists, dentists, nurses, laboratory
technicians and establish rates of pay.

  2. Establish fee schedules for physicians' and dentists' services.

  3. Fix the qualifications for specialists.

  4. Determine the number of individuals for whom any
doctor or dentist may provide service.

  5. Determine what hospitals or clinics may provide service
for patients and under what conditions.

Under the Wagner-Murray-Dingell provisions, it is proposed to:

  1. Appropriate funds for the construction of hospitals and
health facilities.

  2. Provide grants to states for Public Health Services.

  3. Provide grants to states for more comprehensive public
assistance for the needy.

4. Provide grants to states for maternal and child health and welfare services.

5. Provide grants to non-profit corporations and agencies engaged in research or in undergraduate or postgraduate professional education.

6. Reimburse workers during periods of unemployment and for temporary disability.

7. Provide monthly retirement benefits for all male workers having reached the age of 65 and female workers having reached the age of 60.

8. Provide monthly benefits for widows, mothers, parents and dependent children of workers.

9. Provide "Lump Sum Payments" to widows, widowers or heirs on the death of workers.

10. Provide personal health services for all Social Security beneficiaries and their dependents.

Definitions of Personal Health Services in the Wagner-Murray-Dingell provisions:

The General Medical Benefit means services furnished by a legally qualified physician or group of such physicians at the home, office or elsewhere, including diagnostic and therapeutic treatment, care and periodic examination.

The Special Medical Benefit means necessary services requiring special skill or experience by a legally qualified physician who is a specialist or consultant with respect to the class of service furnished.

General Dental Benefit means services furnished by a legally qualified dentist or by a group of such dentists including all necessary dental services and preventive diagnostic and therapeutic treatment, care and advice and periodic examination.

Special Dental Benefit means necessary services requiring special skill or experience, furnished at the office or elsewhere, by a legally qualified dentist who is a specialist or consultant with respect to the class of service furnished.

Home Nursing Benefit means nursing care of the sick, furnished in the home by (1) a registered professional nurse, or (2) a practical nurse who is legally qualified by a state, or (3) who is qualified with respect to standards established by the Surgeon General of the United States Public Health Service.

The opponents of this bill say that if enacted into law and made fully effective it would (1) place all doctors and dentists under direction of a bureaucrat—regiment the medical, dental and nursing professions; (2) destroy the private practice of medicine and dentistry in the United States; (3) inevitably result in a deterioration of the quality of medical and dental care; (4) by a reasonable progression, necessitate the Federal Government conducting the business of producing drugs, pharmaceuticals, eyeglasses, appliances, hospital equipment and supplies; (5) establish a core of collectivist control that surely will be extended and under which free enterprise in any field could not long survive.

The proponents of the Wagner-Murray-Dingell Bill maintain that there will be no deterioration of medical progress in the United States and point to Russia as an example where medical progress has advanced to a very high level under socialized medicine. There may be some restriction to private practice, but it will not be destroyed. It has not been destroyed in Russia where a physician may see a patient and be paid by him for his services while he is being paid by the state at the same time.

It is impossible in this one chapter to review briefly what medicine has done and is doing in the Soviet Union, medicine thoroughly and completely socialized. The reader is referred to the other chapters in this book for the complete story. Medicine in Russia has not been destroyed; it has attained greater heights of achievement than ever before in its history. All the people are the beneficiaries of what medicine and surgery has to offer, not the small number that can afford it.

Socialized medicine is not something that has come into

prominence within recent years. More than fifty years ago Germany instituted by goverment edict a system of sickness insurance for low-income workers. The workers themselves carried two-thirds of the cost and the employers the remainder. This was socialized medicine on a very limited scale. At no time were all, or even a majority of the people provided with medical care.

England has also tried socialized medicine on a small scale. England in 1911 passed the National Insurance Act which made medical care and treatment available to a number of people. But never has it been practiced on as wide a scale as in the Soviet Union.

In the United States various health plans have been in existence for some time now which makes medical care available to people by subscription. Most of the plans are based on the six basic essentials set up by the Committee on the Costs of Medical Care. These are as follows:

1. The plan must safeguard the quality of medical service and preserve the essential personal relation between patient and physician.

2. It must provide for the future development of preventive and therapeutic services in such kinds and amounts as will meet the needs of substantially all the people and not merely present effective demands.

3. It must provide services on financial terms which the people can and will meet, without hardship, through individual or collective resources.

4. There should be a full application of existing knowledge to the prevention of disease so that all medical practice will be permeated with the concept of prevention. The program must include, therefore, not only medical care of the individual and the family, but also a well-organized and adequately supported public health program.

5. The basic plan should include provisions for assisting

and guiding patients in the selection of competent practitioners and suitable facilities for medical care.

6. Adequate and assured payments must be provided to the individuals and agencies which furnish the care.

There are many such organizations throughout the country. In California, for example, the California Medical Association has taken the lead in organizing the California Physicians Service, with over 5,000 physicians as members, to provide medical and hospital care to groups of low or moderate income on a monthly payment basis. This has been a successful venture. Some say that if a government bureaucrat is slipped in between the patient and the doctor, the whole basis of medical practice is changed for the worse. This may be so, but we have not tried this, and until we do, we can never know the answer.

BIBLIOGRAPHY

Asratyan, E. A. "A New Method for the Treatment of Traumatic Shock." *American Review of Soviet Medicine.* October, 1944, p. 37.

Blokhin, N. N. "Skin Plastic Procedures in War Injuries." *Ibid.* December, 1944, p. 104.

Blum, L. L. "Transfusion of Blood and Blood Substitutes in the U.S.S.R." *Ibid.* February, 1945, p. 273.

Bogomolets, A. A. "Anti-Reticular Cytotoxic Serum as a Means of Pathogenetic Therapy." *Ibid.* December, 1943, p. 101.

———. "Blood Transfusion in the Treatment of Internal Diseases." *Ibid.* February, 1945, p. 196.

Borovski, M. L. "The Treatment of Peripheral Nerve Trauma." *Ibid.* June, 1945, p. 543.

Dawson, Percy M. "Physical Culture in the Soviet Union." *Ibid.* October, 1943, p. 48.

Drew, C. R. "The Role of Soviet Investigators in the Development of the Blood Bank." *Ibid.* April, 1944, p. 360.

Filatov, V. P. "Tissue Therapy in Cutaneous Leishmaniasis." *Ibid.* April, 1945, p. 484.

———. "Tissue Therapy in Ophthalmology." *Ibid.* October, 1944, p. 53.

Frumkin, A. P. "Reconstruction of the Male Genitalia." *Ibid.* October, 1944, p. 14.

Gause, G. F. and Brazhnikov, M. G. "Gramicidin S: Its Origin and Mode of Action." *Ibid.* December, 1944, p. 134.

Ginsburg, E. M. "Pathogenesis and Treatment of Lobar Pneumonia." *Ibid.* October, 1944, p. 28.

GIRGOLAV, S. S. "Modern Data on Frostbite." *Ibid.* June, 1945, p. 437.

GOLDBERG, D. I. "The Stimulation of Wound Healing by Embryonal Tissue." *Ibid.* February, 1945, p. 225.

KANSANSKI, V. I. "Frozen Plasma." *Ibid.* February, 1945, p. 207.

———. "Preservation of Erythrocytes and their Clinical Use." *Ibid.* February, 1945, p. 210.

KECHEYEV, K. "The Problem of Night Vision." *Ibid.* April, 1944, p. 300.

KRAVKOV, S. V. "Stimulating Visual Function." *Ibid.* April, 1945, p. 353.

KROTKOV, F. G. "The Use of Greases and Ointments in the Prevention of Frostbite." *Ibid.* June, 1944, p. 443.

KUDRYASHOV, V. A. "Thrombin: Its Properties and Method of Utilization in Surgery." *Ibid.* February, 1945, p. 243.

LEVITIN, F. I. "The Organization of Anti-Tuberculosis Work." *Ibid.* February, 1946, p. 204.

LUKOMSKI, I. "Fluorine in Medicine." *Ibid.* August, 1945, p. 543.

MARCHUK, P. D. "A Method of Preparing and Preserving Anti-Reticular Cytotoxic Serum." *Ibid.* December, 1943, p. 113.

MASHKILLEISON, L. N. and RAKHMANOV, V. A. "Venereal Disease Control in the U.S.S.R." *Ibid.* December, 1945, p. 100.

MITEREV, G. A. "Current Tasks of Public Health." *Ibid.* December, 1945, p. 181.

NEGOVSKI, V. A. "Agonal States and Clinical Death." *Ibid.* August, 1945, p. 491.

PANCHENKO, D. I. "Retrograde Changes in the Spinal Cord in Frostbite of the Extremities." *Ibid.* June, 1944, p. 440.

PINES, L. V. "Certain Mechanisms Involved in Peripheral Nerve Injuries." *Ibid.* December, 1944, p. 149.

PRIOROV, N. N. "The Organization of Traumatologic Services in Soviet Industries." *Ibid.* December, 1944, p. 100.

PROPPER-GRASHSCHENKOV, N. I. "Nerve Transplantation." *Ibid.* October, 1943, p. 28.

——. "The All-Union Institute of Experimental Medicine and the War." *Ibid.* December, 1944, p. 119.

RICKMAN, O. A., OLSHEVSKAYA, V. L. and DIDONOVA, O. N. "Control of Infectious Diseases." *Ibid.* February, 1945, p. 251.

RUSAKOV, A. V. "Wound Pthisis." *Ibid.* December, 1943, p. 145.

SCOTT, J. A. "Venereal Diseases in the Soviet Union." *Ibid.* June, 1945, p. 458.

SERGEYEV, P. "The Struggle Against Malaria." *Ibid.* December, 1945, p. 120.

SERGIEV, P. G. "Gramicidin S in Medical Practice." *Ibid.* December, 1944, p. 143.

SHERSHEVSKAYA, O. I. "Transplantation of the Cornea." *Ibid.* August, 1945, p. 525.

SHIMKIN, M. B. "Experimental Cancer Research in the Soviet Union." *Ibid.* October, 1943, p. 43.

——. "Medical Education in the Soviet Union." *Ibid.* June, 1944, p. 465.

SIGERIST, Henry B. "Medical Care Through Medical Centers in the Soviet Union." *Ibid.* December, 1943, p. 176.

——. "Rural Health Services in the Soviet Union." *Ibid.* February, 1944, p. 270.

SPERANSKY, A. S. "Experimental and Clinical Lobar Pneumonia." *Ibid.* October, 1944, p. 22.

STANLEY, W. M. "Soviet Studies in Viruses." *Ibid.* December, 1943, p. 166.

STERN, Lina S. "A New Method of Treating Tetanus." *Ibid.* August, 1944, p. 540.

WINSLOW, C. E. A. "Public Health in the Soviet Union." *Ibid.* December, 1943, p. 163.

YUDIN, S. S. "Refrigeration Anesthesia for Amputation." *Ibid.* October, 1944, p. 4.

INDEX

274 INDEX